ABC OF BREAST DISEASES

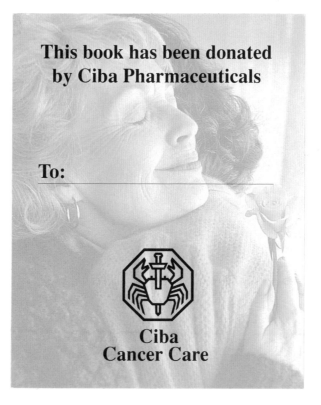

This book has been donated by Ciba Pharmaceuticals

To:

**Ciba
Cancer Care**

ABC OF BREAST DISEASES

edited by
J MICHAEL DIXON
Senior lecturer in surgery, Edinburgh Royal Infirmary and honorary consultant surgeon,
Western General Hospital, Edinburgh

with contributions by

T J ANDERSON, M BAUM, R W BLAMEY, N J BUNDRED, I O ELLIS, R C F LEONARD,
K McPHERSON, P MAGUIRE, R E MANSEL, W R MILLER, D A L MORGAN, D L PAGE,
J PATNICK, M A RICHARDS, D RILEY, A RODGER, J R C SAINSBURY, I E SMITH,
C M STEEL, J D WATSON, A R M WILSON

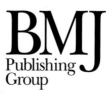
BMJ
Publishing
Group

First published in 1995
by the BMJ Publishing Group, BMA House,
Tavistock Square, London WC1H 9JR

British Library Cataloguing in Publication Data

A catalogue record for this book is available
from the British Library

ISBN 0-7279-0915-0

Typeset in Great Britain by Bedford Typesetters
Printed in Singapore by Craft Print Pte Ltd

Contents

ACKNOWLEDGMENTS

As the diagnosis can often be made by inspection alone, the book is extensively illustrated and I thank the patients whose photographs appear in this book. The speed at which the series in the *BMJ* was produced and the quality of the book owes much to Miss Monica McGill's accurate typing. I thank Deborah Reece and Greg Cotton at the BMJ Publishing Group for their roles in the production of this book. Most of the colour illustrations were prepared by Mr David Dirom of the Medical Illustration and Photographic Unit of the University of Edinburgh. I am grateful to my colleague Mr Udi Chetty, who generously provided a number of colour illustrations. I would like to thank and acknowledge the patience and support of my wife, Pam, and my sons, Oliver and Jonathan, during the months I spent editing the text and checking the proofs. I was generously supported by the Cancer Research Campaign for my first five years as a senior lecturer in the University Department of Surgery, during which time this book was prepared, and I acknowledge their support.

PREFACE

Breast diseases are so common that health professionals in almost every specialty of medicine will be confronted at some time with a patient with a breast disorder. A knowledge of the current investigation and treatment of benign and malignant breast conditions is thus required by a wide range of doctors and ancillary workers in general practice and in different hospital specialties.

Over the past decade there have been significant advances in our understanding of breast disorders, which have led to major changes in both the methods of treatment and the way this treatment is delivered. The *ABC of Breast Diseases* incorporates these advances and presents a succinct, practical account of our current knowledge of benign and malignant breast conditions and their optimal treatment. It reflects the multidisciplinary approach adopted in most breast units and is aimed at all health workers involved in the investigation and treatment of patients with breast disorders.

SYMPTOMS, ASSESSMENT, AND GUIDELINES FOR REFERRAL

J M Dixon, R E Mansel

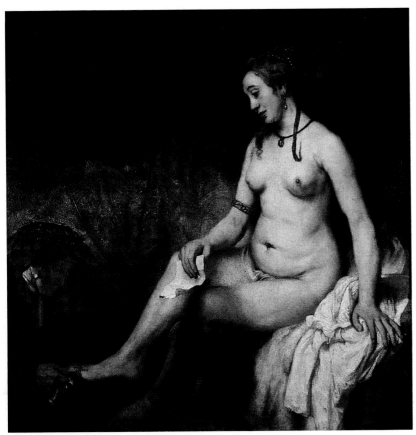

"Bathsheba bathing" by Rembrandt. The model was Rembrandt's mistress, and much discussion has surrounded the shadowing in her left breast and whether this represents an underlying malignancy.

A breast lump, which may be painful, and breast pain constitute over 80% of the breast problems that require hospital referral, and breast problems constitute up to a quarter of the general surgical workload.

Prevalence of presenting symptoms in patients attending a breast clinic	
Breast lump	36%
Painful lump or lumpiness	33%
Pain alone	17·5%
Nipple discharge	5%
Nipple retraction	3%
Strong family history of breast cancer	3%
Breast distortion	1%
Swelling or inflammation	1%
Scaling nipple (eczema)	0·5%

Guidelines for referral to hospital

Conditions that require hospital referral

● All patients with a discrete mass (aspiration of masses by general practitioners is not encouraged, except in patients with a history of multiple breast cysts, because bruising can follow aspiration of a solid mass, making subsequent assessment difficult)

● Nipple discharge in patients aged over 50, and bloodstained, persistent, or troublesome nipple discharge in younger patients

● Mastalgia that interferes with patient's lifestyle or sleep and which has failed to respond to reassurance, simple measures such as wearing a well supporting bra, and common drugs

● Nipple retraction or distortion, change in skin contour, or nipple eczema

● Request for assessment by a patient with a strong family history of breast cancer

● Asymmetrical nodularity that persists at review after menstruation

Patients who can be managed, at least initially, by their general practitioner

● Young patients with tender, lumpy breasts and older patients with symmetrical nodularity, provided that they have no localised abnormality

● Patients with minor and moderate degrees of breast pain who do not have a discrete palpable lesion

● Patients aged under 50 who have nipple discharge that is from more than one duct or is intermittent and is not bloodstained or troublesome

When a patient presents with a breast problem the basic question for the general practitioner is, "Is there a chance that cancer is present, and, if not, can I manage these symptoms myself?"

For patients presenting with a breast lump, the general practitioner should determine whether the lump is discrete or is an area of lumpiness or nodularity. A discrete lump stands out from the adjoining breast tissue, has definable borders, and is measurable. Nodularity is ill defined, often bilateral, and tends to fluctuate with the menstrual cycle.

Assessment of symptoms

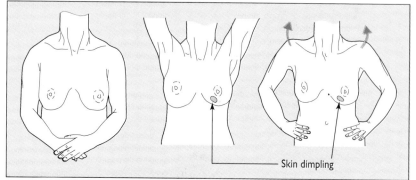

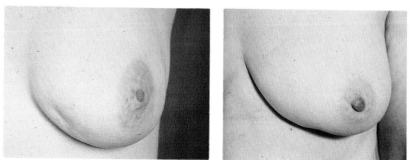

Positions in which breasts should be inspected. Skin dimpling in lower part of breast only evident when arms are elevated or pectoral muscles contracted.

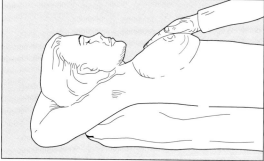

Skin dimpling (left) and change in breast contour (right) associated with underlying breast carcinoma.

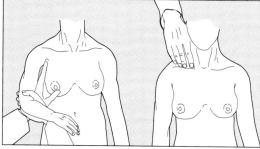

Breast palpation.

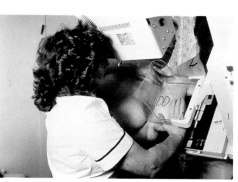

Assessment of regional nodes.

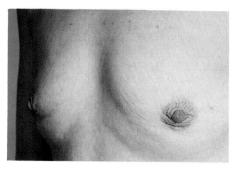

Skin dimpling in both breasts due to breast involution.

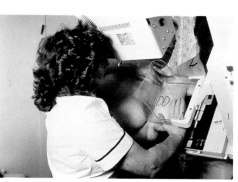

Mammography.

Patient's history

Details of risk factors, including family history and current medication, can be obtained with a simple questionnaire which can be completed by a patient while waiting to be seen in the outpatient clinic. The duration of any symptom is important—breast cancers usually grow slowly, but cysts may appear overnight.

Clinical examination

Inspection should take place in a good light with the patient with her arms by her side, above her head, and pressing on her hips. Skin dimpling or a change in contour is present in a high percentage of patients with breast cancer. Although usually associated with an underlying malignancy, skin dimpling can follow surgery or trauma, be associated with benign conditions, or occur as part of breast involution.

Breast palpation is performed with the patient lying flat with her arms above her head, and all the breast tissue is examined with the hand held flat. Any abnormality should then be further examined with the fingertips and assessed for deep fixation by tensing the pectoralis major—accomplished by asking the patient to press on her hips. All palpable lesions should be measured with callipers.

Assessment of axillary nodes—Once both breasts have been palpated the nodal areas are checked. Clinical assessment of axillary nodes is often inaccurate: palpable nodes can be identified in up to 30% of patients with no clinically significant breast or other disease, and up to 40% of patients with breast cancer who have clinically normal axillary nodes actually have axillary nodal metastases.

Mammography

Mammography requires compression of the breast between two plates and is uncomfortable. Single views of each breast can be taken obliquely, or two views—oblique and craniocaudal—can be obtained. With modern film screens a dose of less than 1·5 mGy is standard. Mammography allows detection of mass lesions, areas of parenchymal distortion and microcalcifications. Because breasts are relatively radiodense in women aged under 35, mammography is rarely of value in this age group.

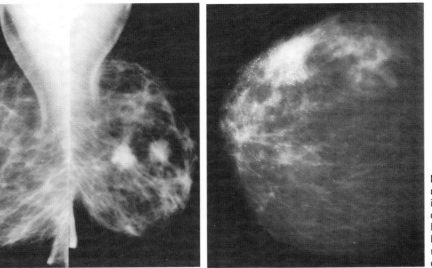

Mammograms showing (left) two mass lesions in left breast irregular in outline with characteristics of carcinomas, and (right) a mass lesion with the extensive, branching, impalpable microcalcification characteristic of carcinoma in situ.

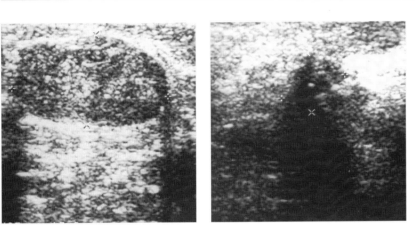

Ultrasound scans showing clear edges of fibroadenoma (left) and indistinct outline of carcinoma (right).

Ultrasonography

High frequency sound waves are beamed through the breast, and reflections are detected and turned into images. Cysts show up as transparent objects, and other benign lesions tend to have well demarcated edges whereas cancers usually have indistinct outlines.

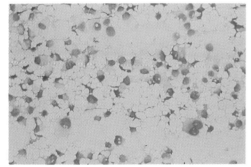

Cell smear showing malignancy—cancer cells are lying singly, and they and their nuclei vary substantially in size and shape.

Fine needle aspiration cytology

Needle aspiration can differentiate between solid and cystic lesions. Aspiration of solid lesions requires skill to obtain sufficient cells for cytological analysis, and expertise is needed to interpret the smears. In a few centres cytopathologists take the specimens, but aspirations are usually performed by a clinician. A 21 or 23 gauge needle is attached to a syringe, which is used with or without a syringe holder. The needle is introduced into the lesion and suction is applied by withdrawing the plunger; multiple passes are made through the lesion. The plunger is then released, and the material is spread onto microscope slides. These are then either air dried or sprayed with a fixative, depending on the cytologist's preference, and are later stained. In some units a report is available within 30 minutes.

Core biopsy

A small core is removed from the mass by means of a cutting needle technique. Several needles are available, and some can be combined with mechanical devices to allow the procedure to be performed single handed.

Open biopsy

Open biopsy should be performed only in patients who have been appropriately investigated by imaging, fine needle aspiration cytology, and, if appropriate, core biopsy. Women who are told that investigations have shown their lesion to be benign rarely request excision.

Breast biopsy is not without morbidity. A fifth of patients develop either a further lump under the scar or pain specifically related to the biopsy site.

Indications for excision of breast lesion

- Diagnosis of malignancy on cytology that is not supported by results of other investigations when a mastectomy or axillary clearance is planned
- Suspicion of malignancy on one or more investigations even when other investigations indicate that lesion is probably benign
- Request by patient for excision
- Some units excise all symptomatic discrete breast masses in patients aged over 40

Symptoms, assessment, and guidelines for referral

> **The routine use of frozen section to diagnose breast cancer is no longer acceptable**

> Other techniques such as computed tomography, magnetic resonance imaging, thermography, radioisotope studies, nipple cytology, and ductography have no role in routine investigation of patients with breast problems

Frozen section

Frozen section should be used only in the following circumstances:
- Confirmation of a cytological diagnosis of malignancy before proceeding to definitive surgery (such patients should already have been told that their lesion is malignant and have been appropriately counselled, with discussion of all treatment options)
- Assessment of excision margins for a wide local excision to ensure complete excision
- Assessment of axillary nodes to identify patients who are node negative and who require only a limited dissection

Accuracy of investigations

> ### Accuracy of investigations in diagnosis of symptomatic breast disease in specialist breast clinics
>
> | | Clinical examination | Mammography | Ultrasonography | Fine needle aspiration cytology |
> |---|---|---|---|---|
> | Sensitivity for cancers* | 86% | 86% | 82% | 95% |
> | Specificity for benign disease† | 90% | 90% | 85% | 95% |
> | Positive predictive value for cancers‡ | 95% | 95% | 90% | 99·8% |
>
> *% Of cancers detected by test as malignant or probably malignant (that is, complete sensitivity).
> †% Of benign disease detected by test as benign.
> ‡% Of lesions diagnosed as malignant by test that are cancers (that is, absolute positive predictive value).

False positive results occur with all diagnostic techniques. It is now routine to plan treatment on the basis of malignant cytology supported by a diagnosis of malignancy on clinical examination and imaging. Cytology has a false positive rate of about two per 1000, and the lesions most likely to be misinterpreted are fibroadenomas and areas of breast that have been irradiated. The sensitivity of clinical examination and mammography varies with age, and only two thirds of cancers in women aged under 50 are deemed suspicious or definitely malignant on clinical examination or mammography.

Triple assessment

Triple assessment is the combination of clinical examination, imaging (mammography for women aged 35 or over and ultrasonography for women aged under 35), and fine needle aspiration cytology. In a recent series of 1511 patients with breast cancer having triple assessment, only six patients (0·2%) had lesions that were considered to be benign on all three investigations.

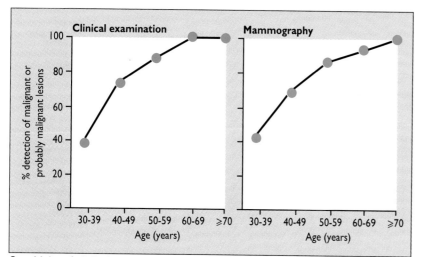

Sensitivity of clinical examination and mammography by age in patients presenting with a breast mass.

Advantages and disadvantages of techniques for assessment of breast masses

Technique	Advantages	Disadvantages
Clinical examination	Easy to perform	Low sensitivity in women aged ≤50
Mammography	Useful for screening women aged ≥50	Requires dedicated equipment and experienced personnel Low sensitivity in women aged ≤50 Unpleasant (causes discomfort or actual pain)
Ultrasonography	Same sensitivity in all ages Useful in assessing impalpable lesions Painless	Operator dependent Less sensitive and less specific than clinical examination or mammography
Fine needle aspiration cytology	Cheap High sensitivity Provides definitive diagnosis in most instances Low incidence of false positives	Operator dependent Needs experienced cytopathologist Painful

Investigation of breast symptoms

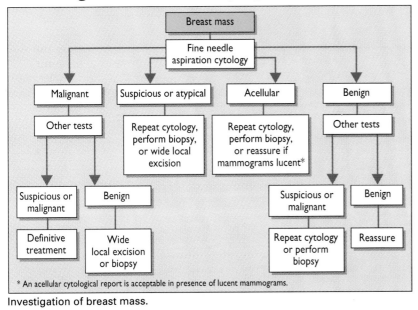

* An acellular cytological report is acceptable in presence of lucent mammograms.

Investigation of breast mass.

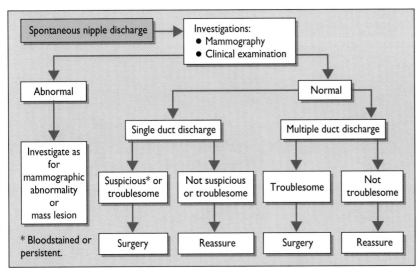

* Bloodstained or persistent.

Investigation of nipple discharge.

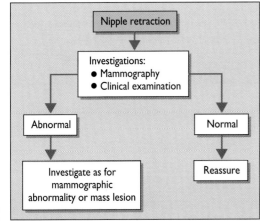

Investigation of nipple retraction.

Breast mass

All patients should be assessed by triple assessment. It is not necessary to excise all solid breast masses, and a selective policy is recommended based on the results of triple assessment.

Nipple discharge

Treatment depends on whether the discharge is spontaneous and whether it is from one or several ducts. If the discharge is red or brown in colour the presence of blood should be checked by testing for haemoglobin. All patients with spontaneous discharge should have clinical examination and, if aged over 35, mammography. Physiological nipple discharge is common: two thirds of premenopausal women can be made to produce nipple secretion by cleansing the nipple and applying suction. This physiological discharge varies in colour from white to yellow to green to blue-black.

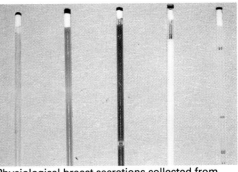

Physiological breast secretions collected from non-pregnant women. Note range of colours from white to blue-black.

Nipple retraction

Slit-like retraction of the nipple is characteristic of benign disease whereas nipple inversion, when the whole nipple is pulled in, occurs in association with both breast cancer and inflammatory breast conditions.

Breast pain

Cyclical breast pain should be differentiated from non-cyclical pain, and its severity should be assessed by means of a careful history and a pain chart. Mammography or ultrasonography is indicated in patients with either unilateral persistent mastalgia or localised areas of painful nodularity. Focal lesions should be investigated with fine needle aspiration cytology.

The painting by Rembrandt is reproduced by permission of the Bridgeman Art Library.

CONGENITAL PROBLEMS AND ABERRATIONS OF NORMAL BREAST DEVELOPMENT AND INVOLUTION

J M Dixon, R E Mansel

Congenital abnormalities

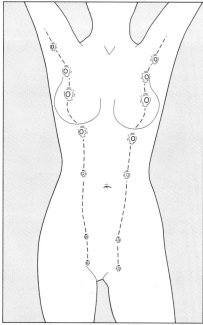

Usual sites of accessory nipples and breasts along milk lines.

Extra nipples and breasts

Between 1% and 5% of men and women have supernumerary or accessory nipples or, less frequently, supernumerary or accessory breasts. These usually develop along the milk line: the most common site for accessory nipples is just below the normal breast, and the most common site for accessory breast tissue is the lower axilla. Accessory breasts below the umbilicus are extremely rare. Extra breasts or nipples rarely require treatment unless unsightly, although they are subject to the same diseases as normal breasts and nipples.

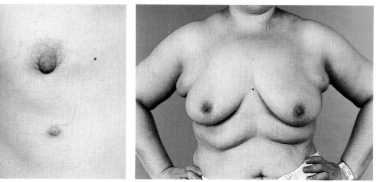

Patients with an accessory nipple (left) and bilateral accessory breasts (right).

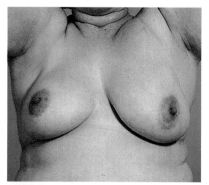

Left breast hypoplasia.

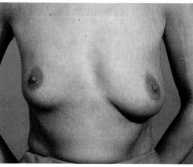

Breast asymmetry.

Absence or hypoplasia of the breast

One breast can be absent or hypoplastic, usually in association with defects in pectoral muscle. Some degree of breast asymmetry is usual, and the left breast is more commonly larger than is the right. True breast asymmetry can be treated by augmentation of the smaller breast, reduction or elevation of the larger breast, or a combination of procedures.

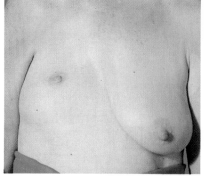

Absence of right pectoralis major muscle but normal right breast.

Poland's syndrome with hypoplasia of right breast and absent chest wall muscles. (Patient also had typical hand abnormality.)

Chest wall abnormalities

About 90% of patients with true unilateral absence of a breast have either absence or hypoplasia of the pectoral muscles. In contrast, 90% of patients with pectoral muscle defects have normal breasts. Some patients have abnormalities of the pectoral muscles and absence or hypoplasia of the breast associated with a characteristic deformity of the upper limb. This cluster of anomalies is called Poland's syndrome. Abnormalities of the chest wall, such as pectus excavatum, and deformities of the thoracic spine can also result in normal symmetrical breasts seeming asymmetrical.

Breast development and involution

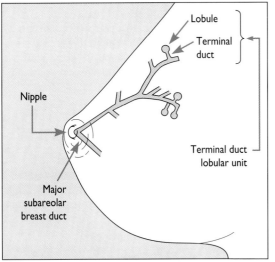

Anatomy of breast showing terminal duct lobular units and branching system of ducts.

The breast is identical in boys and girls until puberty. Growth begins at about the age of 10 and may initially be asymmetrical: a unilateral breast lump in a 9-10 year old girl is invariably developing breast, and biopsy specimens should not be taken from girls of this age as they can damage the breast bud. The functional unit of the breast is the terminal duct lobular unit or lobule, which drains via a branching duct system to the nipple. The duct system does not run in a truly radial manner, and the breast is not separated into easily defined segments. The lobules and ducts—the glandular tissue—are supported by fibrous tissue—the stroma. Most benign breast conditions and almost all breast cancers arise within the terminal duct lobular unit.

Aberrations of normal breast development and involution

Age (years)	Normal process	Aberration
<25	Breast development	
	Stromal	Juvenile hypertrophy
	Lobular	Fibroadenoma
25-40	Cyclical activity	Cyclical mastalgia Cyclical nodularity (diffuse or focal)
35-55	Involution	
	Lobular	Macrocysts
	Stromal	Sclerosing lesions
	Ductal	Duct ectasia

After the breast has developed, it undergoes regular changes in relation to the menstrual cycle. Pregnancy results in a doubling of the breast weight at term, and the breast involutes after pregnancy. In nulliparous women breast involution begins at some time after the age of 30. During involution the breast stroma is replaced by fat so that the breast becomes less radiodense, softer, and ptotic (droopy). Changes in the glandular tissue include the development of areas of fibrosis, the formation of small cysts (microcysts), and an increase in the number of glandular elements (adenosis). The life cycle of the breast consists of three main periods: development (and early reproductive life), mature reproductive life, and involution. Most benign breast conditions occur during one specific period and are so common that they are best considered as aberrations rather than disease.

Aberrations of breast development

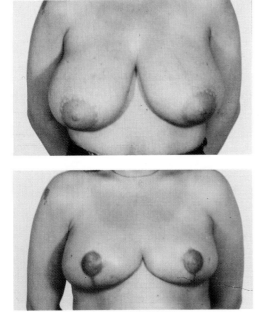

Patient with juvenile hypertrophy (top) and after surgery (bottom).

Juvenile or virginal hypertrophy

Prepubertal breast enlargement is common and only requires investigation if it is associated with other signs of sexual maturation. Uncontrolled overgrowth of breast tissue can occur in adolescent girls whose breasts develop normally during puberty but then continue to grow, often quite rapidly. No endocrine abnormality can be detected in these girls.

Patients present with social embarrassment, pain, discomfort, and inability to perform regular daily tasks. Reduction mammoplasty considerably improves their quality of life and should be more widely available.

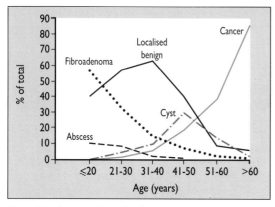

Changing frequencies of different discrete breast lumps with age.

Fibroadenoma

Although classified in most textbooks as benign neoplasms, fibroadenomas are best considered as aberrations of normal development: they develop from a whole lobule and not from a single cell, they are very common, and they are under the same hormonal control as the remainder of the breast tissue. They account for about 13% of all palpable symptomatic breast masses, but in women aged 20 or less they account for almost 60% of such masses. There are four separate types of fibroadenoma: common fibroadenoma, giant fibroadenoma, juvenile fibroadenoma, and phyllodes tumours. There is no universally accepted definition of what constitutes a giant fibroadenoma, but most consider that it should measure over 5 cm in diameter. Juvenile fibroadenomas occur in adolescent girls and sometimes undergo rapid growth but are managed in the same way as the common fibroadenoma. Phyllodes tumours are distinct pathological entities and cannot always be clinically differentiated from fibroadenomas.

A definitive diagnosis of fibroadenoma can be made by a combination of clinical examination, ultrasonography, and fine needle aspiration cytology. They have characteristic mammographic features in older patients when they calcify, and a few patients have multiple fibroadenomas. Current evidence of the natural course of fibroadenomas suggests that less than 10% of them increase in size and about one third get smaller or completely disappear.

Management—Fibroadenomas over 4 cm in diameter should be excised. In women aged under 40 fibroadenomas diagnosed by clinical examination, ultrasonography, and fine needle aspiration cytology do not need excision unless this is requested by the patient. In women aged over 40 a selective policy of excision should be used to ensure that breast cancers are not missed.

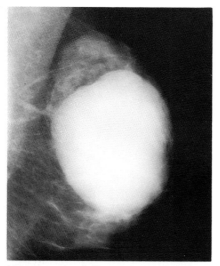

Juvenile fibroadenoma of right breast.

Aberrations in early reproductive period

Final diagnosis in patients with palpable breast mass

Localised benign*	38%
Carcinoma	26%
Cysts	15%
Fibroadenoma	13%
Periductal mastitis	1%
Duct ectasia	1%
Abscess	1%
Others	5%

*Localised areas of nodularity that histologically show no clinically significant abnormality or aberrations of normal involution

Pain and nodularity

Cyclical pain and nodularity are so common that they can be regarded as physiological and not pathological. Pain which is severe or prolonged is regarded as an aberration. Focal breast nodularity is the most common cause of a breast lump and is seen in women of all ages. When excised most of these areas of nodularity show either no pathological abnormality or aberrations of the normal involutional process such as focal areas of fibrosis or sclerosis. The preferred pathological term is benign breast change, and terms such as fibroadenosis, fibrocystic disease, and mastitis should no longer be used by clinicians or pathologists.

Aberrations of involution

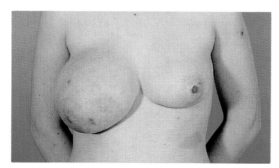

Mammogram of discrete breast lesion with surrounding halo characteristic of breast cyst.

Cystic disease

This term should be restricted to the clearly defined group of women with a palpable breast cyst. Cystic disease affects 7% of women in Western countries, and cysts constitute 15% of all discrete breast masses. Cysts are distended and involuted lobules and are seen most frequently in perimenopausal women. Most present as a smooth discrete breast lump that can be painful and is sometimes visible.

Cysts have characteristic halos on mammography and are readily diagnosed by ultrasonography. The diagnosis is established by needle aspiration, and providing the fluid is not bloodstained it should not be sent for cytology. After aspiration the breast should be re-examined to check that the palpable mass has disappeared. Any residual mass requires full assessment by mammography and fine needle aspiration cytology as 1-3% of patients with cysts have carcinomas; few of these are associated with a cyst.

Patients with multiple cysts have a slightly increased risk of developing breast cancer, but the magnitude of this risk is not considered of clinical significance.

Congenital problems and aberrations of normal breast development and involution

Sclerosis

Aberrations of stromal involution include the development of localised areas of excessive fibrosis or sclerosis. Pathologically, these lesions can be separated into three groups: sclerosing adenosis, radial scars, and complex sclerosing lesions (this term incorporates lesions previously called sclerosing papillomatosis or duct adenoma and includes infiltrating epitheliosis).

These lesions are of clinical importance because of the diagnostic problems they cause during breast screening. Excision biopsy is often required to make a definitive diagnosis.

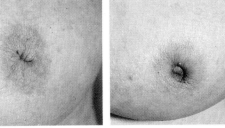

Slit-like nipple retraction due to duct ectasia (left) and nipple retraction due to breast cancer (right).

Duct ectasia

The major subareolar ducts dilate and shorten during involution, and, by the age of 70, 40% of women have substantial duct dilatation or duct ectasia. Some women with excessive dilatation and shortening present with nipple discharge, nipple retraction, or a palpable mass that may be hard or doughy. The discharge is usually cheesy, and the nipple retraction is classically slit-like. Surgery is indicated if the discharge is troublesome or the patient wishes the nipple to be everted.

Epithelial hyperplasia

Epithelial hyperplasia is an increase in the number of cells lining the terminal duct lobular unit. This was previously called epitheliosis or papillomatosis, but these terms are now obsolete. The degree of hyperplasia can be graded as mild, moderate, or florid.

If the hyperplastic cells also show cellular atypia the condition is called atypical hyperplasia. The absolute risk of breast cancer developing in a woman with atypical hyperplasia who does not have a first degree relative with breast cancer is 8% at 10 years: for a woman with a first degree relative with breast cancer, the risk is 20-25% at 15 years.

Gynaecomastia

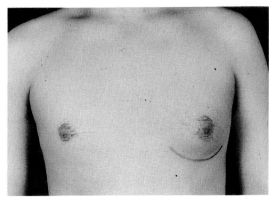

Patient with left sided gynaecomastia. Black line indicates lower limit of dissection.

Gynaecomastia (the growth of breast tissue in males to any extent in all ages) is entirely benign and usually reversible. It commonly occurs in puberty and old age. It is seen in 30-60% of boys aged 10-16 years and usually requires no treatment as 80% resolve spontaneously within two years. Embarrassment or persistent enlargement are indications for surgical referral.

Senescent gynaecomastia commonly affects men aged between 50 and 80, and in most it does not appear to be associated with any endocrine abnormality. A careful history and examination will often reveal the cause. A history of recent progressive breast enlargement without pain or tenderness and without an easily identifiable cause is an indication for investigation. Mammography can differentiate between breast enlargement due to fat or gynaecomastia and is of value if malignancy is suspected. Fine needle aspiration cytology should be performed if there is clinical or mammographic suspicion of breast cancer. Only if no clear cause is apparent should blood hormone concentrations be measured.

In drug related gynaecomastia withdrawal of the drug or change to an alternative treatment should be considered. Gynaecomastia is seen increasingly in body builders who take anabolic steroids; some have learnt that by taking tamoxifen they can combat this. Danazol produces symptomatic improvement in some patients with gynaecomastia.

Causes of gynaecomastia

Puberty	25%
Idiopathic (senescent)	25%
Drugs (cimetidine, digoxin, spironolactone, androgens, or antioestrogens)	10-20%
Cirrhosis or malnutrition	8%
Primary hypogonadism	8%
Testicular tumours	3%
Secondary hypogonadism	2%
Hyperthyroidism	1·5%
Renal disease	1%

Benign neoplasms

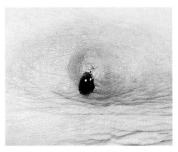

Bloodstained nipple discharge.

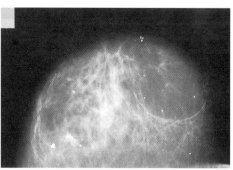

Mammogram showing a large radiolucent lipoma present anteriorly and medially in breast. (White mark represents lateral aspect of mammogram.)

Duct papillomas

These can be single or multiple. They are very common, and it has been suggested that they should be considered as aberrations rather than true benign neoplasms since they show minimal malignant potential. The most common symptom is nipple discharge, which is often bloodstained.

Lipomas

These soft lobulated radiolucent lesions are common in the breast. Interest in these lesions lies in the confusion with pseudo-lipoma, a soft mass that can be felt around a breast cancer and which is caused by indrawing of the surrounding fat by a spiculated carcinoma.

There are other benign tumours that occur in the breast, but these are rare.

BREAST PAIN

R E Mansel

Breast pain (mastalgia) alone or in association with lumpiness is reported in up to a half of all women attending breast clinics. Two thirds of a group of working women and 77% of a screening population admitted to having had recent breast pain when directly questioned. Most mastalgia is of minor or moderate severity and is accepted as part of the normal changes that occur in relation to the menstrual cycle. Studies have clearly shown that women who complain of mastalgia are psychologically no different from women attending hospital outpatient clinics for other conditions.

> Breast pain of any type is a rare symptom of breast cancer, and only 7% of patients with breast cancer have mastalgia as their only symptom

Classification

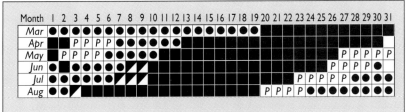

Daily breast pain chart.

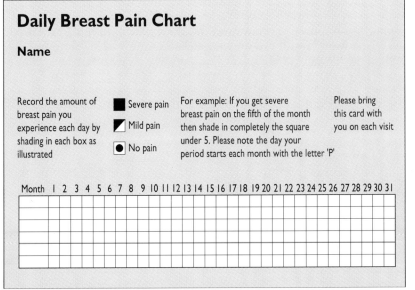

Breast pain chart of patient with severe cyclical mastalgia. (P indicates menstrual period.)

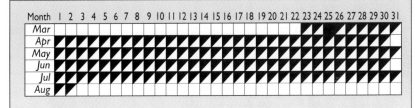

Breast pain chart of patient with moderate continuous non-cyclical mastalgia.

Breast pain can be separated into two main groups, cyclical and non-cyclical. The best way to assess whether pain is cyclical is to ask a patient to complete a breast pain record chart. Two thirds of women have cyclical pain, and the remaining third have non-cyclical pain.

Cyclical mastalgia

Patients with cyclical pain are by definition premenopausal, and their average age is 34. Normal changes in relation to menstrual cycle are heightened awareness, discomfort, fullness, and heaviness of the breast during the three to seven days before each period. Women often report areas of tender lumpiness in their breasts and increased breast size at this time. Patients with cyclical mastalgia typically suffer increasing severity of pain from mid-cycle onwards, with the pain improving at menstruation. The pain is usually described as heavy with the breast being tender to touch, and it classically affects the outer half of the breast. The pain varies in severity from cycle to cycle but can persist for many years.

Cyclical mastalgia is relieved by the menopause, but pregnancy, oral contraceptives, and parity do not affect its course. Physical activity can increase the pain: this is particularly relevant for women whose occupations include lifting and prolonged use of the arms. The impact of mastalgia on quality of life is often underestimated.

Non-cyclical mastalgia

This affects older women (mean age 43). The pain can arise from the chest wall, the breast itself, or outside the breast. Non-cyclical mastalgia may be continuous but is usually described as having a random time pattern; the pain is often localised and described as a "burning" or "drawing."

Breast pain
Assessment of patients

A careful history is necessary to exclude non-breast conditions. Clinical examination must be performed to exclude a clinically important mass lesion in the breast. If no mass is identified further investigation is not indicated and the patient should be reassured that there is no sinister cause for her symptoms. The impact of the pain on the patient's quality of life should then be determined. Severe mastalgia tends to interfere with work, hugging children, and sexual relationships. If treatment is being considered patients should be asked to complete a pain chart for at least two months to allow identification of the pattern of pain and to assess the number of days of pain in each menstrual cycle.

Aetiology

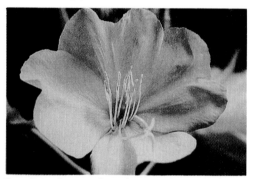

Evening primrose *Oenothera erythrosepala* is a perennial herb that takes its name from its unusual habit of opening its flowers between six and seven o'clock in the evening. The plant is rich in an oil containing the essential fatty acid γ-linolenic acid (gamolenic acid).

Despite the close temporal relation with the menstrual cycle, hormonal studies have failed to reveal any clear differences in patients with mastalgia, although a few reports indicate that there may be a slight elevation of prolactin stores (as measured with the thyrotrophin releasing hormone stimulation test). Women with mastalgia have also been found to have abnormal plasma fatty acid profiles, but the role of dietary factors such as caffeine and fats in the aetiology of breast pain is unclear. An abnormal profile of certain essential fatty acids might explain the response of breast pain to agents such as evening primrose oil. Many women with cyclical mastalgia report breast swelling and abdominal bloating in the luteal phase of their menstrual cycles, but studies measuring total body water show no difference between patients with mastalgia and controls: this is consistent with the observation that diuretic treatment is of no value in mastalgia.

Treatment

Response of cyclical and non-cyclical mastalgia to drug treatment

	Useful response to treatment		
	Cyclical mastalgia	Non-cyclical mastalgia	Side effects
Danazol	79%	40%	30%
Gamolenic acid	58%	38%	4%
Bromocriptine	54%	33%	35%

Drawbacks and side effects of drugs to treat mastalgia
Gamolenic acid
- Mild nausea
- Slow response to treatment

Danazol
- Weight gain
- Acne
- Hirsutism

Bromocriptine
- Nausea
- Dizziness

Cyclical breast pain

The primary indication for treatment is pain which interferes with everyday activities. Many women who present to hospital do so because they are worried that mastalgia may indicate breast cancer. Reassurance that cancer is not responsible for their symptoms and an explanation of the hormonal basis of the pain are the only treatment necessary in up to 85% of women with cyclical mastalgia. Some women can improve their pain with simple measures such as wearing a soft support sleep bra at night.

Many general practitioners still use antibiotics for mastalgia: these are ineffective and should be used only when a specific diagnosis of periductal mastitis or lactational infection has been made. Diuretics and vitamin B-6 have not been shown to be of value in cyclical mastalgia. Progestogens have been used both orally and topically and are ineffective. Some patients who are taking an oral contraceptive find that their breast pain improves after stopping the pill and changing to mechanical contraception, but no individual oral contraceptive has been shown to specifically cause mastalgia. Premenopausal women who start hormone replacement therapy often report an increase in breast pain and nodularity, which usually settles with continued therapy.

There are presently three drugs that can be prescribed for cyclical mastalgia. Patients with moderate pain and those who wish to continue taking oral contraceptives should first be given evening primrose oil (prescribed as capsules containing gamolenic acid 40 mg, six to eight to be taken daily in divided doses). This drug has only minor side effects, and, as the reaction to therapy can be slow, a trial of treatment should last at least four months. The effects of treatment can be monitored with pain charts.

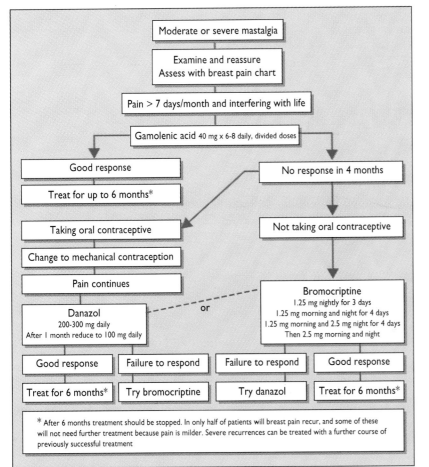

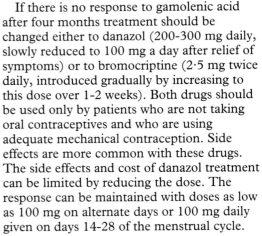

Protocol for treating moderate to severe cyclical mastalgia. (Mild mastalgia requires examination and reassurance.)

If there is no response to gamolenic acid after four months treatment should be changed either to danazol (200-300 mg daily, slowly reduced to 100 mg a day after relief of symptoms) or to bromocriptine (2·5 mg twice daily, introduced gradually by increasing to this dose over 1-2 weeks). Both drugs should be used only by patients who are not taking oral contraceptives and who are using adequate mechanical contraception. Side effects are more common with these drugs. The side effects and cost of danazol treatment can be limited by reducing the dose. The response can be maintained with doses as low as 100 mg on alternate days or 100 mg daily given on days 14-28 of the menstrual cycle.

Responses to danazol and bromocriptine are usually seen within three months. If there is no response to one of these three drugs it is worth trying one of the other agents: second or third line responses occur in about 30% of patients. If the outlined treatment plan is followed about 70-80% of patients should experience substantial relief of symptoms. Other drugs such as tamoxifen and goserelin (a gonadotrophin releasing hormone agonist) are effective in treating cyclical mastalgia but are not currently licensed for this condition in the United Kingdom.

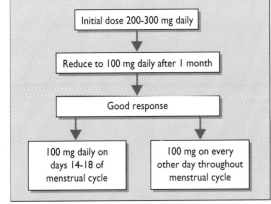

Protocol for reducing dosage of danazol.

Classification of non-cyclical mastalgia

Chest wall causes
- For example, tender costochondral junctions (Tietze's syndrome)

True breast pain
- Diffuse breast pain
- Trigger spots in breast

Non-breast causes
- Cervical and thoracic spondylosis
- Bornholm disease
- Lung disease
- Gall stones
- Exogenous oestrogens such as hormone replacement therapy
- Thoracic outlet syndrome

Non-cyclical mastalgia

Localised pain in the chest wall, referred pain, and diffuse true breast pain must be differentiated. Appropriate treatment should be started for referred pain. Up to 60% of patients with a persistent localised painful area in the chest wall can be effectively treated by infiltration with local anaesthetic and steroid injection (2 ml of 1% lignocaine combined with 40 mg of methylprednisolone in 1 ml). Injection of local anaesthetic confirms the correct identification of the painful area by producing complete disappearance of the pain.

Wearing a firm supporting bra 24 hours a day often improves true non-cyclical breast pain. True diffuse breast pain should be treated initially with a non-steroidal anti-inflammatory drug. If this fails some women respond to the drugs used for cyclical mastalgia. Because of its low incidence of side effects gamolenic acid should be the first of these agents to be tried.

Some women have a localised single tender area in the breast, which is known as a trigger spot. Some of these respond to injection of local anaesthetic and steroid. It has been reported that pain can be eliminated in up to half of these women by excision of the trigger spot. However, surgery generally makes breast pain worse—some women develop non-cyclical breast pain at the site of previous breast operations. Excision of tender painful areas in an attempt to relieve symptoms is therefore rarely appropriate.

BREAST INFECTION

J M Dixon

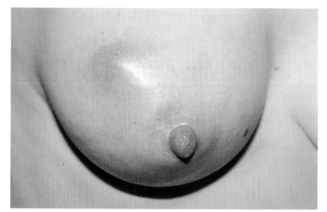

A breast abscess which developed during breast feeding.

Organisms responsible for breast infections	
Type of breast infection	Organism
Neonatal	*Staphylococcus aureus* (*Escherichia coli*)*
Lactating	*Staphylococcus aureus* (*Staphylococcus epidermidis*)* (*Streptococci*)*
Non-lactating	*Staphylococcus aureus* Enterococci Anaerobic streptococci *Bacteroides* spp
Skin associated	*Staphylococcus aureus* (*Fungi*)*

*Organisms only occasionally responsible.

Breast infection is now much less common than it used to be. It is seen occasionally in neonates, but it most commonly affects women aged between 18 and 50; in this age group it can be divided into lactational and non-lactational infection. The infection can affect the skin overlying the breast, when it can be a primary event, or it may occur secondary to a lesion in the skin such as a sebaceous cyst or to an underlying condition such as hidradenitis suppurativa.

Treatment

Antibiotics most appropriate for treating breast infections*		
Type of breast infection	No allergy to penicillin	Allergy to penicillin
Neonatal, lactating, and skin associated	Flucloxacillin (500 mg four times daily)	Erythromycin (500 mg twice daily)
Non-lactating	Co-amoxiclav (375 mg thrice daily)	Combination of cephradine (500 mg four times daily) or erythromycin (500 mg twice daily) with metronidazole (200 mg thrice daily)

*Doses are for adults.

There are four guiding principles in treating breast infection
- Appropriate antibiotics should be given early to reduce formation of abscesses
- Hospital referral is indicated if the infection does not settle rapidly with antibiotics
- If an abscess is suspected it should be confirmed by aspiration before it is drained surgically
- Breast cancer should be excluded in patients with an inflammatory lesion which is solid on aspiration or which does not settle despite apparently adequate treatment

All abscesses in the breast can be managed by repeated aspiration or incision and drainage. Few breast abscesses require drainage under general anaesthesia except those in children, and placement of a drain after incision and drainage is unnecessary.

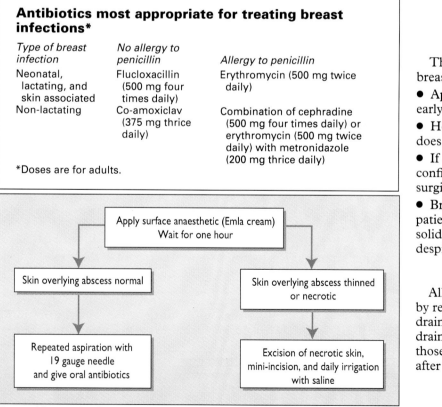

Protocol for treating breast abscesses.

Neonatal infection

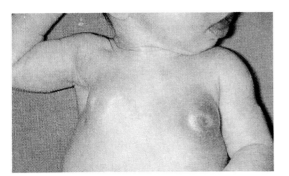

Neonatal breast abscess.

Neonatal breast infection is most common in the first few weeks of life when the breast bud is enlarged. Although *Staphylococcus aureus* is the usual organism, *Escherichia coli* is occasionally the pathogen. If an abscess develops the incision to drain the pus should be placed as peripheral as possible to avoid damaging the breast bud.

Lactating infection

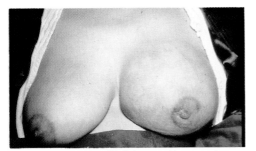

Puerperal mastitis of left breast. Note erythema, oedema, and obvious signs of inflammation, especially medially.

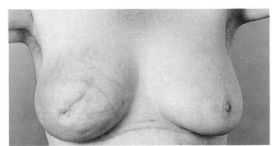

Inflammatory carcinoma of right breast. Note erythema and peau d'orange.

Better maternal and infant hygiene and early treatment with antibiotics have considerably reduced the incidence of abscess formation during lactation. Infection is most frequently seen within the first six weeks of breast feeding, although some women develop it with weaning. Lactating infection presents with pain, swelling, and tenderness. There is usually a history of a cracked nipple or skin abrasion. *Staphylococcus aureus* is the most common organism responsible, but *S epidermidis* and streptococci are occasionally isolated. Drainage of milk from the affected segment should be encouraged and is best achieved by continuing breast feeding. Tetracycline, ciprofloxacin, and chloramphenicol should not be used to treat lactating breast infection as they may enter breast milk and can harm the baby.

If the infection does not settle after a course of flucloxacillin and no pus is obtained on aspiration but the cytology indicates the lesion is infective or inflammatory, the antibiotic should be changed to co-amoxiclav to cover other possible pathogens. If the inflammation or an associated mass lesion still persists then further investigations are required to exclude an underlying carcinoma. An established abscess should be treated by either recurrent aspiration or incision and drainage. Many women wish to continue to breast feed, and they should be encouraged to do so.

Non-lactating infection

Non-lactating infections can be separated into those occurring centrally in the periareolar region and those affecting the peripheral breast tissue.

Periareolar infection

Periareolar infection is most commonly seen in young women with a mean age of 32. Histologically, there is active inflammation around non-dilated subareolar breast ducts—a condition termed periductal mastitis. This condition has been confused with and called duct ectasia, but duct ectasia is almost certainly a separate condition affecting an older age group and characterised by subareolar duct dilatation and less pronounced and less active periductal inflammation. Current evidence suggests that smoking is an important factor in the aetiology of periductal mastitis but not in duct ectasia: about 90% of women who get periductal mastitis or its complications smoke cigarettes compared with 38% of the same age group in the general population. Substances in cigarette smoke may either directly or indirectly damage the wall of the subareolar breast ducts. The damaged tissues then become infected by either aerobic or anaerobic organisms. Initial presentation may be with periareolar inflammation (with or without an associated mass) or with an established abscess. Associated features include central breast pain, nipple retraction at the site of the diseased duct, and nipple discharge.

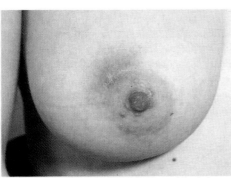

Periareolar inflammation due to periductal mastitis. Minor degree of nipple retraction present at site of diseased duct.

Breast infection

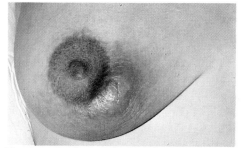

Non-lactating breast abscess due to periductal mastitis. Nipple retracted towards site of infection at areolar margin.

Treatment—A periareolar inflammatory mass should be treated with a course of appropriate antibiotics, and abscesses should be managed by aspiration or incision and drainage. Care should be taken to exclude an underlying neoplasm if the mass or inflammation does not resolve after appropriate treatment. Abscesses associated with periductal mastitis commonly recur because treatment by incision or aspiration does not remove the underlying diseased duct. Up to a third of patients develop a mammary duct fistula after drainage of a non-lactating periareolar abscess. Recurrent episodes of periareolar sepsis should be treated by excision of the diseased duct under antibiotic cover by an experienced breast surgeon.

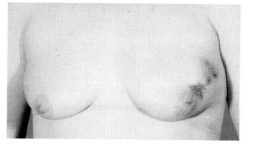

Diagram of mammary duct fistula with arrow showing path of fistula probe. Dots around left hand duct represent periductal mastitis, a precursor of a fistula.

Mammary duct fistula

A mammary duct fistula is a communication between the skin usually in the periareolar region and a major subareolar breast duct. A fistula can develop after incision and drainage of a non-lactating abscess, it can follow spontaneous discharge of a periareolar inflammatory mass, or it can result from biopsy of a periductal inflammatory mass.

Treatment is by excision of the fistula and diseased duct or ducts under antibiotic cover. Recurrence is common after surgery, and the lowest rates of recurrence and best cosmetic results have been achieved in specialist breast units.

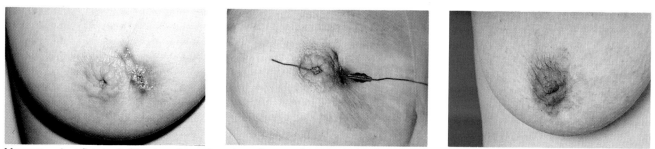

Mammary duct fistula: (left) external opening at areolar margin and whole of nipple inverted; (centre) probe passed through opening of fistula and emerging from affected duct; and (right) after excision of fistula and affected duct and primary wound closure under antibiotic cover. Operation performed through a circumareolar incision, which gives an excellent cosmetic result.

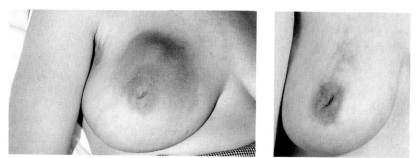

Granulomatous lobular mastitis of left breast. Multiple scars and nipple retraction.

Peripheral breast abscess before management (left) and after recurrent aspiration and oral antibiotics (right).

Peripheral non-lactating breast abscesses

These are less common than periareolar abscesses and are often associated with an underlying condition such as diabetes, rheumatoid arthritis, steroid treatment, granulomatous lobular mastitis, and trauma. Pilonidal abscesses in sheep shearers and barbers have been reported to occur in the breast. Infection associated with granulomatous lobular mastitis can be a particular problem. This condition affects young parous women, who may develop large areas of infection with multiple simultaneous peripheral abscesses. There is a strong tendency for this condition to persist and recur after surgery. Large incisions and extensive surgery should therefore be avoided in this condition. Steroids have been tried but with limited success. Peripheral breast abscesses should be treated by recurrent aspiration or incision and drainage.

Skin associated infection

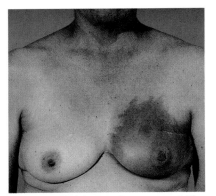

Cellulitis of left breast that occurred 18 months after left wide local excision and radiotherapy.

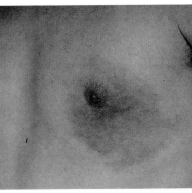

Cellulitis of left breast of adolescent male.

Primary infection of the skin of the breast, which can present as cellulitis or an abscess, most commonly affects the skin of the lower half of the breast. These infections are often recurrent in women who are overweight, have large breasts, or have poor personal hygiene. Cellulitis most commonly affects the skin of the breast after surgery or radiotherapy. *Staphylococcus aureus* is the usual causative organism, although fungal infections have been reported. Cellulitis in the male breast is uncommon but is seen in the neonatal and pubertal periods.

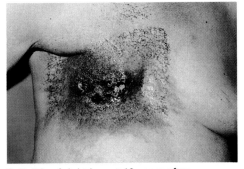

Cellulitis of right breast 10 years after mastectomy, prosthesis insertion, and radiotherapy. Areas of ulceration are due to erosion of prosthesis through the skin. The wound settled and healed after treatment with co-amoxiclav.

Treatment of acute bacterial infection is with antibiotics and drainage or aspiration of abscesses. Women with recurrent infections should be advised about weight reduction and keeping the area as clean and dry as possible (this includes careful washing of the area up to twice a day, avoiding skin creams and talcum powder, and wearing either a cotton bra or a cotton T shirt or vest worn inside the bra.

Sebaceous cysts are common in the skin of the breast and may become infected. Some recurrent infections in the inframammary fold are due to hidradenitis suppurativa. In this condition the infection should first be controlled by a combination of appropriate antibiotics and drainage of any pus (the same organisms are found in hidradenitis as in non-lactating infection). Conservative excision of the affected skin is effective at stopping further infection in about half of patients; the remainder have further episodes of infection despite surgery.

Other infections and conditions

Tuberculosis of the breast is now rare and can be primary or, more commonly, secondary. Clues to its diagnosis include the presence of a breast or axillary sinus in up to half of patients. The commonest presentation of tuberculosis nowadays is with an abscess resulting from infection of a tuberculous cavity by an acute pyogenic organism such as *Staphylococcus aureus*. An open biopsy is often required to establish the diagnosis. Treatment is by a combination of surgery and antituberculous chemotherapy.

Syphilis, actinomycosis, and mycotic, helminthic, and viral infections occasionally affect the breast but are rare.

Factitial disease

Artefactual or factitial diseases are created by the patient, often through complicated or repetitive actions. Such patients may undergo many investigations and operations before the nature of the disease is recognised. The diagnosis is difficult to establish but should be considered when the clinical situation does not conform to common appearances or pathological processes.

Tuberculosis of left breast with multiple sinuses.

BREAST CANCER—EPIDEMIOLOGY, RISK FACTORS, AND GENETICS

K McPherson, C M Steel, J M Dixon

Worldwide incidence of cancers in women (1980)

Site of cancer	No of cases (1000s)	% Of total
Breast	572	18
Cervix	466	15
Colon and rectum	286	9
Stomach	261	8
Endometrium	149	5
Lung	147	5
Ovary	138	4
Mouth and pharynx	121	4
Oesophagus	108	4
Lymphoma	98	3

Computer enhanced mammogram of a breast cancer.

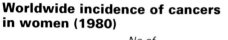

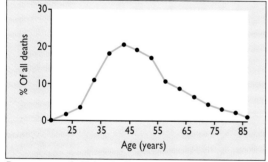

Percentage of all deaths in women attributable to breast cancer.

With 570 000 new cases in the world each year, breast cancer remains the commonest malignancy in women and comprises 18% of all female cancers. In the United Kingdom, where the age standardised incidence and mortality is the highest in the world, the incidence among women aged 50 approaches two per 1000 women per year, and the disease is the single commonest cause of death among women aged 40-50, accounting for about a fifth of all deaths in this age group. There are more than 15 000 deaths each year, and the incidence is increasing slowly, particularly among elderly women, by about 1-2% a year.

Of every 1000 women aged 50, two will recently have had breast cancer diagnosed and about 15 will have had a diagnosis made before the age of 50, giving a prevalence of breast cancer of nearly 2%.

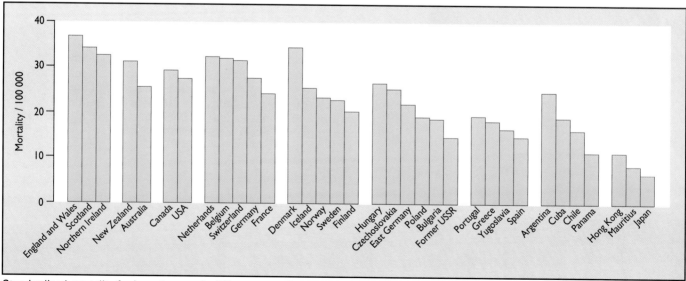

Standardised mortality for breast cancer in different countries.

Risk factors for breast cancer

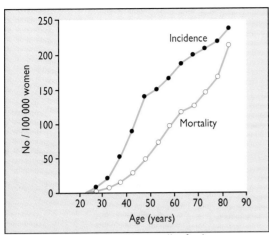

Age specific incidence and mortality for breast cancer in United Kingdom.

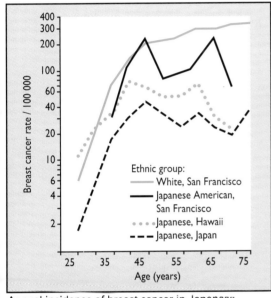

Annual incidence of breast cancer in Japanese women in Japan, Hawaii, and San Francisco and in white women from San Francisco.

Established and probable risk factors for breast cancer

Factor	Relative risk	High risk group
Age	>10	Elderly
Geographical location	5	Developed country
Age at menarche	3	Menarche before age 11
Age at menopause	2	Menopause after age 54
Age at first full pregnancy	3	First child in early 40s
Family history	≥2	Breast cancer in first degree relative when young
Previous benign disease	4-5	Atypical hyperplasia
Cancer in other breast	>4	
Socioeconomic group	2	Groups I and II
Diet	1·5	High intake of saturated fat
Body weight:		
Premenopausal	0·7	Body mass index >35
Postmenopausal	2	Body mass index >35
Alcohol consumption	1·3	Excessive intake
Exposure to ionising radiation	3	Abnormal exposure in young females after age 10
Taking exogenous hormones:		
Oral contraceptives	2	Use for ≥4 years when young
Hormone replacement therapy	1·5	Use for ≥10 years
Diethylstilbestrol	2	Use during pregnancy

Age

The incidence of breast cancer increases with age, doubling about every 10 years until the menopause, when the rate of increase slows dramatically. Compared with lung cancer, the incidence of breast cancer is higher at younger ages. In some countries there is a flattening of the age-incidence curve after the menopause.

Geographical variation

Age adjusted incidence and mortality for breast cancer varies by up to a factor of seven between countries. The difference between Far Eastern and Western countries is diminishing but is still about fivefold. Studies of migrants from Japan to Hawaii show that the rates of breast cancer in migrants assume the rate in the host country within one or two generations, indicating that environmental factors are of greater importance than genetic factors.

Age at menarche and menopause

Women who start menstruating early in life or who have a late menopause have an increased risk of developing breast cancer. Women who have a natural menopause after the age of 55 are twice as likely to develop breast cancer as women who experience the menopause before the age of 45. At one extreme, women who undergo bilateral oophorectomy before the age of 35 have only 40% of the risk of breast cancer of women who have a natural menopause.

Age at first pregnancy

Nulliparity and late age at first birth both increase the lifetime incidence of breast cancer. The risk of breast cancer in women who have their first child after the age of 30 is about twice that of women who have their first child before the age of 20. The highest risk group are those who have a first child after the age of 35; these women appear to be at even higher risk than nulliparous women. An early age at birth of a second child further reduces the risk of breast cancer.

Family history

Up to 10% of breast cancer in Western countries is due to genetic predisposition. Breast cancer susceptibility is generally inherited as an autosomal dominant with limited penetrance. This means that it can be transmitted through either sex and that some family members may transmit the abnormal gene without developing cancer themselves. It is not yet known how many breast cancer genes there may be. About a third of the familial cases are thought to be due to mutations in the BRCA1 gene on the long arm of chromosome 17. This gene has just been cloned, and preliminary reports suggest that it is a large gene and that mutations are not confined to particular regions. Some inherited BRCA1 mutations may be associated with different risks of breast cancer. A second hereditary breast cancer locus, BRCA2, has been identified on the long arm of chromosome 13. In addition, a few cases arise from mutations in the p53 gene on the short arm of chromosome 17.

Breast cancer—epidemiology, risk factors, and genetics

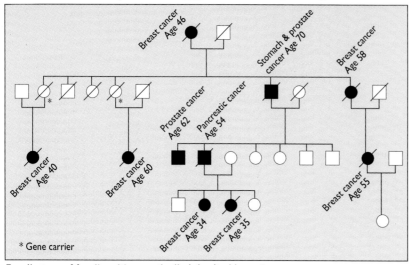

Many families affected by breast cancer show an excess of ovarian, colon, prostatic, and other cancers attributable to the same inherited mutation. Patients with bilateral breast cancer, those who develop a combination of breast cancer and another epithelial cancer, and women who get the disease at an early age are most likely to be carrying a genetic mutation that has predisposed them to developing breast cancer. Most breast cancers that are due to a genetic mutation occur before the age of 65, and a woman with a strong family history of breast cancer of early onset who is still unaffected at 65 has probably not inherited the genetic mutation.

Family tree of family with genetically inherited breast cancer.

A woman's risk of breast cancer is two or more times greater if she has a first degree relative (mother, sister, or daughter) who developed the disease before the age of 50, and the younger the relative when she developed breast cancer the greater the risk. For example, a woman whose sister developed breast cancer aged 30-39 has a cumulative risk of 10% of developing the disease herself by age 65, but that risk is only 5% (close to the population risk) if the sister was aged 50-54 at diagnosis. The risk increases by between four and six times if two first degree relatives develop the disease. For example, a woman with two affected relatives, one who was aged under 50 at diagnosis, has a 25% chance of developing breast cancer by the age of 65.

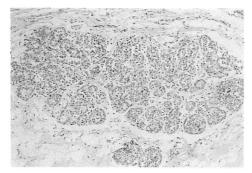

Severe atypical lobular hyperplasia.

Previous benign breast disease

Women with severe atypical epithelial hyperplasia have a four to five times higher risk of developing breast cancer than women who do not have any proliferative changes in their breast. Women with this change and a family history of breast cancer (first degree relative) have a ninefold increase in risk. Women with palpable cysts, complex fibroadenomas, duct papillomas, sclerosis adenosis, and moderate or florid epithelial hyperplasia have a slightly higher risk of breast cancer (1·5-2 times) than women without these changes, but this increase is not clinically important.

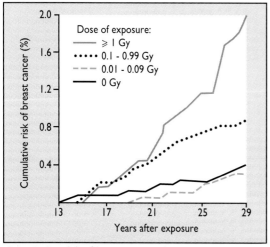

Cumulative risk of breast cancer in women who were aged 10-19 years when exposed to radiation from atomic bombs during second world war.

Radiation

A doubling of risk of breast cancer was observed among teenage girls exposed to radiation during the second world war. Ionising radiation also increases risk later in life, particularly when exposure is during rapid breast formation. Mammographic screening is associated with a net decrease in mortality from breast cancer among women aged over 50; the effect of such exposure on younger women remains unclear.

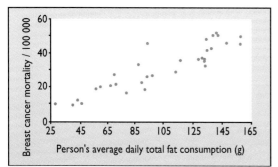

Relation between breast cancer mortality in various countries and fat consumption.

Lifestyle

Diet—Although there is a close correlation between the incidence of breast cancer and dietary fat intake in populations, the true relation between fat intake and breast cancer does not appear to be particularly strong or consistent.

Weight—Obesity is associated with a twofold increase in the risk of breast cancer in postmenopausal women whereas among premenopausal women it is associated with a reduced incidence.

Alcohol intake—Some studies have shown a link between alcohol consumption and incidence of breast cancer, but the relation is inconsistent and the association may be with other dietary factors rather than alcohol.

Smoking is of no importance in the aetiology of breast cancer.

Relative risk of breast cancer before menopause in relation to use of oral contraceptives before first term pregnancy	
Length of use (months)	Relative risk (95% confidence interval)
0	1
1-24	1·04 (0·9 to 1·2)
25-48	1·21 (1·0 to 1·5)
49-96	1·34 (1·1 to 1·6)
>96	1·61 (1·2 to 2·2)

Oral contraceptive

There is no increase in risk in women who have used oral contraceptives in their late 20s for spacing pregnancies. However, use of oral contraceptives for four years or more by younger women before their first term pregnancy almost certainly increases the risk of premenopausal breast cancer. Whether such women also have an increased risk of postmenopausal breast cancer will not be known until exposed women achieve that age. Studies of nulliparous users of oral contraceptives indicate that there may be an effect on early stage carcinogenesis, which would not be evident for a considerable period. This was the situation for women exposed to diethylstilbestrol while pregnant during the 1940s and '50s, with the increased risk of breast cancer not becoming apparent until 20 to 40 years after exposure. Since use of oral contraceptives by young women was not common until the 1970s, data on any association with risk of breast cancer remain immature.

Hormone replacement therapy

Studies of unopposed oestrogen for hormone replacement therapy show that the risk of breast cancer is increased by up to 50% after 10 to 15 years' use. This effect is less than an equivalent natural delay in the menopause. Fewer data are available on the use of combined oestrogen and progestogen preparations, but the only large study published to date shows a greater risk for the combined treatment than for unopposed therapy. The benefits of hormone replacement therapy in reducing ischaemic heart disease and osteoporosis and improving menopausal symptoms suggest that for the first 10 years of use the overall effects of therapy on morbidity and mortality are likely to be beneficial. One problem is that breast density can increase with hormone replacement therapy, which can make detection of breast cancers more difficult.

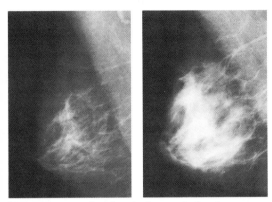

Mammograms of patient before and after three years of hormone replacement therapy showing increase in density caused by treatment.

Prevention of breast cancer

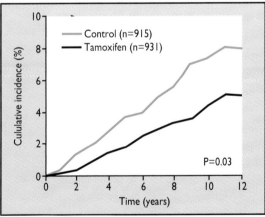

Cumulative incidence of contralateral breast cancer in randomised trial of adjuvant tamoxifen treatment.

The sources of the data presented in illustrations are: J Buell, *J Natl Cancer Inst* 1973;**51**:1479-83 for the graph of incidence of cancer in Japanese migrants; L J Kinlen, *Br Med Bull* 1991;**47**:462-9 (copyright British Council) for the graph of relation between cancer mortality and fat consumption; M Tokunaga *et al*, *J Natl Cancer Inst* 1979;**62**:1347-59 for the graph of risk of cancer after exposure to radiation; Delgado-Rodriguez, *Fertility Reviews* 1992;**1**:22-3 for the table of relation of cancer with use of oral contraceptives; and L E Rutqvist *et al*, *J Natl Cancer Inst* 1991;**83**:1299-306 for the graph of trial of adjuvant tamoxifen treatment. The data are reproduced with permission of the journals or copyright holders.

Screening as it is currently practised can reduce mortality but not incidence, and then only in a particular age group, and advances in treatment have produced only modest survival benefits. A better appreciation of factors important in the aetiology of breast cancer would raise the possibility of disease prevention.

Hormonal control—One promising avenue for primary prevention is influencing the hormonal milieu of women at risk. During trials of tamoxifen as an adjuvant treatment for breast cancer, the number of contralateral breast cancers was less than expected, suggesting that this drug might have a role in preventing breast cancer. Studies comparing tamoxifen with placebo in women at high risk of breast cancer are currently under way, but results from such prevention trials will need to be interpreted cautiously. It is clear that tamoxifen will probably reduce the initial incidence of breast cancer, but only if there is a consequent reduction in mortality will we know that tamoxifen is effective in reducing the number of breast cancers developing rather than just delaying their presentation.

Dietary intervention—If specific dietary factors are found to be associated with an increased risk of breast cancer dietary intervention will be possible. However, reduction of dietary intake of such a factor in whole communities may well be difficult to achieve without major social and cultural changes.

Other preventive agents—Retinoids affect the growth and differentiation of epithelial cells, and experiments suggest that they may have a role in preventing breast cancer. A clinical trial of a retinoid is currently under way. Selenium is another possible cancer preventing agent.

SCREENING FOR BREAST CANCER

R W Blamey, A R M Wilson, J Patnick

> **The aim of screening is to detect breast cancer when it is small and before it has had the chance to spread**

Lack of knowledge of the pathogenesis of breast cancer means that primary prevention is currently a distant prospect. Screening represents an alternative approach to try to reduce mortality from breast cancer.

Methods of screening

There is no evidence that clinical examination, breast ultrasonography, and teaching self examination of the breast are effective tools in screening for breast cancer. Randomised controlled trials have shown, however, that screening by mammography can significantly reduce mortality from breast cancer. Mortality can be reduced by up to 40% in women who attend for screening, and the benefit is greatest in women aged over 50. Published data from the combined Swedish trials showed an overall reduction in breast cancer mortality of 29% during 12 years of follow up in women aged over 50 who were invited to attend screening and a 13% reduction in younger women.

Screening tests should be simple to apply, cheap, easy to perform, easy and unambiguous to interpret, and able to identify women with disease and exclude those without disease. Mammography is expensive; it requires high technology machinery, special film and dedicated processing, and highly trained radiologists to interpret the films; and it detects only 95% of all breast cancers. It is, however, the best screening tool available for detecting breast cancer and is the only screening method for any malignancy which has been shown to be of value in randomised trials.

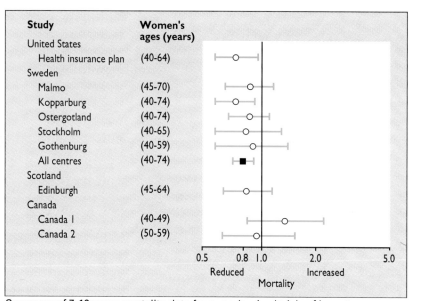

Summary of 7-12 years mortality data from randomised trials of breast cancer screening. Points and lines represent absolute change in mortality and confidence interval.

Organisational aspects of screening

> **Organisation of screening**
> - Accurate population lists
> - Encouragement by general practitioners to attend
> - Clear screening protocols
> - Agreed patterns of referral
> - Well trained assessment team
> - Built in quality assurance
> - Continual audit and education

Over 70% of the target population must accept the invitation to participate if a screening programme is to significantly reduce mortality. If fewer participate the costs per life year saved rises and, although some will clearly benefit, the cost effectiveness of the programme comes into question. To achieve this, accurate lists of names, ages, and current addresses are required. Factors affecting attendance for screening include encouragement to attend by patients' general practitioners, knowledge about the screening programme, and the views of family and friends. Screening programmes should include both the initial screening process and assessment of any abnormality detected.

Standards should be set to ensure quality assurance at each stage of the screening process. Protocols should include referral for treatment to teams experienced in the management of breast disease. Specific training and programmes of continuing education related to screening should be mandatory for all professionals involved in the programme. Regular audit and review of both individual and programme results are essential.

Recommendations for screening

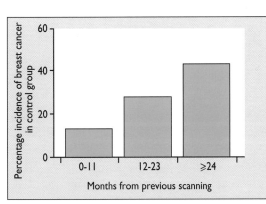

Rates of interval cancer after a negative screen in women aged 50-69.

Age range

Current data indicate that the reduction in mortality is greatest in women aged 50-70. Although data from the combined Swedish trials show a reduction in mortality in younger women, the reduction is not significant and is delayed by at least eight years. Currently, therefore, there is no evidence to support screening of women aged under 50.

Frequency of screening

The most appropriate interval between mammographic screens has yet to be determined. From a cost-benefit point of view, screening once every three years for women aged 50-64 appears to be the optimal screening policy. However, the rate of interval cancer climbs rapidly between the second and third years after the initial screen, suggesting that a three year interval is too long. The best frequency for screening is probably between 18 months and two years.

Number of mammographic views

Whether patients should be screened initially by a single oblique mammogram or have two view mammography is not clear. Proponents of two view mammography argue that the extra expense of taking two x ray pictures is offset by an increase in the rate of detecting breast cancer and a reduction in recall rates. Two views do, however, double the radiation dose. For second and subsequent screens a single view is sufficient.

The basic screen

Detection of breast cancer in women aged 50-64 after an initial screen

	No of women
Initial screen	10 000
Recalled for assessment	<700
Biopsy required	<100
Breast cancer detected	60

The first part of screening is the basic screen. A radiologist is responsible for ensuring appropriate levels of sensitivity and specificity. Among women aged 50-64, at least 50 cancers should be detected for every 10 000 attenders at an initial screen, reflecting the prevalence of cancer (currently the British programme detects over 60 per 10 000). At the subsequent screens 35 cancers should be identified for every 10 000 attenders, reflecting the incidence of cancer. Recall rates for assessment should be below 7% after initial screens and 3% after subsequent screens; many units are recalling fewer than 3·5% after initial screens and 1·5% after subsequent screens. Women who are not found to have any important abnormality should be informed of their "normal" result within two weeks. Patients judged to have an important abnormality require further assessment.

Assessment

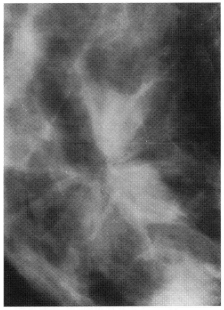

Impalpable stellate lesion detected by screening. Lesion is either a radial scar or an invasive carcinoma, and so excision is required even if results of cytology or core biopsy are reported as benign.

There are two end points to assessment: no important abnormality or a diagnosis of breast cancer. Assessment requires further imaging and sometimes also clinical examination and cytology (triple assessment). Assessments are best performed by a dedicated assessment team consisting of an experienced radiologist, surgeon, and pathologist supported by a breast care nurse.

About two thirds of screen detected abnormalities are shown to be unimportant on further mammographic or ultrasound scanning. Counselling from a breast care nurse may be useful for women with a normal outcome, and it is mandatory for women who require further assessment or treatment for suspected or proved malignancy. In patients with important lesions the aim is to achieve a specific diagnosis by fine needle aspiration cytology or core needle biopsy. When the results of all investigations are available they are discussed by the multidisciplinary team, and a management decision is taken. Fine needle aspiration cytology can confirm a benign process and can definitively establish malignancy, allowing a full discussion with a patient of the diagnosis and treatment options. Any surgery thereafter can be definitive. A biopsy should be performed if there is a suspicion of malignancy on either radiological or clinical grounds even when the results of cytology or core biopsy are benign.

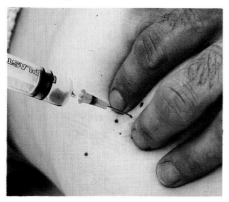

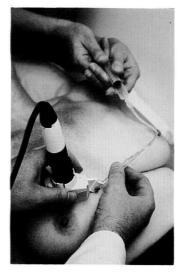

Fine needle aspiration: performed freehand (above) and guided by ultrasound image (right).

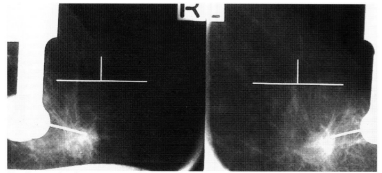

Radiographs for stereotactic guided fine needle aspiration. Needle can be seen penetrating the lesion.

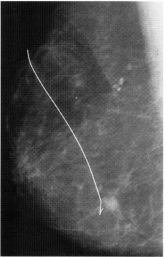

Mammogram after placement of hooked wire adjacent to mammographic lesion.

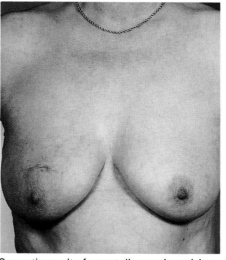

Cosmetic result of recent diagnostic excision biopsy—small scar and no loss of tissue.

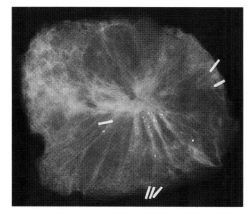

Specimen radiograph of therapeutic excision showing wide clearance margins around impalpable lesion. Ligaclips aid orientation—1 anterior, 2 medial, 3 inferior.

Palpable lesions

Fine needle aspiration of palpable lesions is usually carried out freehand or can be image guided if there is doubt that the palpable lesion coincides with the radiological abnormality. Image guided aspiration is of value if the first freehand aspiration fails to achieve a definitive diagnosis. There may be advantages to having the results of fine needle aspiration cytology reported immediately.

Impalpable lesions

Up to 70% of important abnormalities detected by screening are impalpable, and image guided fine needle aspiration is necessary. Impalpable lesions may be localised by ultrasonography if visible on this modality or by mammography. Ultrasonography is more accurate, quicker, easier to perform, cheaper, and associated with less patient discomfort. Some impalpable lesions— including most microcalcifications, several architectural disturbances, and some stellate lesions—are not visible on ultrasound scans and require x ray guided needle aspiration or core biopsy. Stereotaxis is the most accurate of the x ray guided techniques; cytology should be performed with a 22 or 23 gauge needle of 9 cm length and core biopsy with a 14 gauge needle.

Wire localisation biopsy and excision

Ultrasonography and stereotaxis can facilitate surgery of impalpable lesions that require excision by allowing placement of a hooked wire adjacent to the mammographic lesion. The surgeon can follow the wire when making the incision and then excise breast tissue adjacent to the hook. Accurate placement of the wire is essential, and a variety of wire systems are available.

If the procedure is being performed to establish a diagnosis, a small representative portion of the lesion is excised through a small incision, so leaving a satisfactory cosmetic result if the lesion proves to be benign (according to surgical quality assurance guidelines the biopsy specimen should weigh less than 20 g). In therapeutic excisions (lesions diagnosed by cytology or core biopsy to be malignant or highly suspicious of malignancy) the lesions should be widely excised with a 10-15 mm margin of normal tissue. Intraoperative specimen radiology is essential, both to check that the impalpable lesion has been removed and, if cancer has been diagnosed, to ensure that an adequate wide local excision has been performed.

Benefits and potential drawbacks of screening

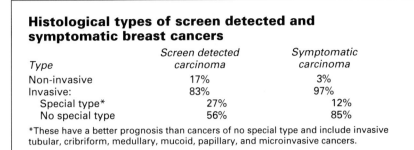

Histological types of screen detected and symptomatic breast cancers

Type	Screen detected carcinoma	Symptomatic carcinoma
Non-invasive	17%	3%
Invasive:	83%	97%
Special type*	27%	12%
No special type	56%	85%

*These have a better prognosis than cancers of no special type and include invasive tubular, cribriform, medullary, mucoid, papillary, and microinvasive cancers.

Characteristics of screen detected cancers

Compared with symptomatic cancers, screen detected cancers are smaller and more likely to be non-invasive (in situ), while any invasive cancers detected are more likely to be better differentiated, of special type, and node negative. The ability of screening to influence mortality from breast cancer indicates that early diagnosis identifies breast cancers at an earlier stage in their evolution when the chances of metastatic disease being present is smaller.

Psychological morbidity induced by screening

No increase in anxiety has been found in women invited to attend breast screening. There does appear to be a short term increase in anxiety associated with recall for assessment, but, by three months after attending for assessment, women who are shown to have no important abnormality (false positives) are no more anxious than control women. It has been suggested that the excess years as a breast cancer patient caused by a cancer being diagnosed earlier might diminish a patient's quality of life, but the psychological morbidity in women with screen detected breast cancer has been reported to be similar to or less than that in age matched controls.

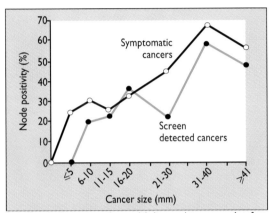

Relation between node positivity and tumour size for screen detected and symptomatic breast cancers.

Risks of mammography

It has been calculated that for every two million women aged over 50 who have been screened by means of a single mammogram one extra cancer a year after 10 years may be caused by the radiation delivered to the breast. Compared with an incidence of breast cancer that approaches 2000 in every million women aged 60, this risk is very small.

Overdiagnosis of breast cancer

Some of the small, well differentiated, invasive cancers and some in situ cancers that are detected by screening would almost certainly not have caused symptoms during the patient's lifetime. However, results from the Swedish randomised trials indicate that the number of breast cancers that are being overdiagnosed by screening is small.

Observed and expected detection of invasive cancer at initial screening of Swedish women aged 50-69

No of cancers detected

Observed	Expected
291	321·6

Unnecessary biopsies

A proportion of women who undergo biopsy will be found not to have cancer, but in Britain the number of women undergoing a biopsy for benign disease is small. The proportion of benign biopsies performed in a screening programme should be monitored and compared with that in an unscreened group of women of the same age. Women who require biopsy are likely to be extremely anxious, but there is no evidence that this anxiety is sustained if the results are benign.

Results from breast screening in Scotland 1991-2

No of women screened	91 028
No of women recalled	6 667 (7·3%)
No of biopsies performed	794
No of cancers detected	578
Biopsy rate*	8·7
Cancer detection rate*	6·3
Benign biopsy rate*	2·4
Ratio of malignant to benign biopsy	2·6:1

*Per 1000 women screened.

The sources of the data presented in illustrations are: J M Dixon and J R C Sainsbury, *Handbook of Diseases of the Breast* (Churchill Livingstone) 1993:86 for the graph of results of trials of screening; L Tabar *et al*, *Br J Cancer* 1987;55:547-51 for the graph of rates of interval cancers between screens; T J Anderson *et al*, *Br J Cancer* 1991;64:108-13 for the graph of node positivity and cancer size for screen detected and symptomatic cancers; and N E Day, *Br Med Bull* 1991;47:400-17 (copyright British Council) for the table of observed and expected detection of cancer by screening. The data are reproduced with permission of the journals or copyright holders.

BREAST CANCER

J R C Sainsbury, T J Anderson, D A L Morgan

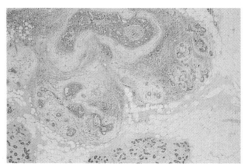

Breast cancers are derived from the epithelial cells that line the terminal duct lobular unit. Cancer cells that remain within the basement membrane of the elements of the terminal duct lobular unit and the draining duct are classified as in situ or non-invasive. An invasive breast cancer is one in which there is dissemination of cancer cells outside the basement membrane of the ducts and lobules into the surrounding adjacent normal tissue. Both in situ and invasive cancers have characteristic patterns by which they can be classified.

Carcinoma in situ affecting a breast lobule.

Classification of invasive breast cancers

Classification of invasive breast cancers

Special types

- Tubular ● Cribriform ● Medullary
- Mucoid ● Papillary ● Classic Lobular

No special type

- Commonly known as NST or NOS (not otherwise specified)
- Useful prognostic information can be gained by grading such cancers

The most commonly used classification of invasive breast cancers divides them into ductal and lobular types. This classification was based on the belief that ductal carcinomas arose from ducts and lobular carcinomas from lobules. We now know that invasive ductal and lobular breast cancers both arise from the terminal duct lobular unit, and this terminology is no longer appropriate. Some tumours show distinct patterns of growth and cellular morphology, and on this basis certain types of breast cancer can be identified. Those with specific features are called invasive carcinomas of special type, while the remainder are considered to be of no special type. This classification has clinical relevance in that certain special type tumours have a much better prognosis than tumours that are of no special type.

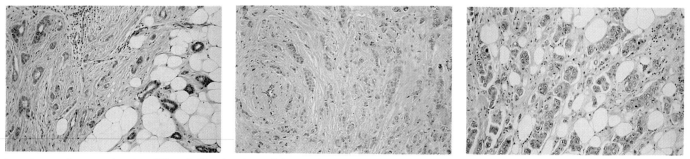

Invasive carcinomas showing diffuse infiltration through breast tissue: grade I (left), grade II (centre), and grade III (right).

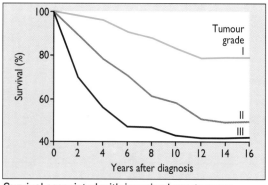

Survival associated with invasive breast cancer according to tumour grade.

Tumour differentiation

Among the cancers of no special type, prognostic information can be gained by grading the degree of differentiation of the tumour. Degrees of glandular formation, nuclear pleomorphism, and frequency of mitoses are scored from 1 to 3. For example, a tumour with many glands would score 1 whereas a tumour with no glands would score 3. These values are combined and converted into three groups: grade I (score 3-5), grade II (scores 6 and 7), and grade III (scores 8 and 9). This derived histological grade—often known as the Bloom and Richardson grade or the Scarff, Bloom, and Richardson grade after the originators of this system—is an important predictor of both disease free and overall survival.

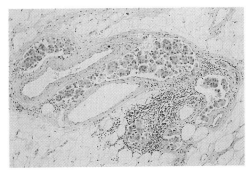

Tumour cells in lymphatic or vascular space.

Other features

Other histological features in the primary tumour are also of value in predicting local recurrence and prognosis.

Lymphatic or vascular invasion—The presence of cancer cells in blood or lymphatic vessels is a marker of more aggressive disease, and patients with this feature are at increased risk of both local and systemic recurrence.

Extensive in situ component—If more than 25% of the main tumour mass contains non-invasive disease and there is in situ cancer in the surrounding breast tissue the cancer is classified as having an extensive in situ component. Patients with such tumours are more likely to develop local recurrence after breast conserving treatment.

Staging of invasive breast cancers

TNM classification of breast tumours

T_{is}	Cancer in situ
T_1	≤2 cm (T_{1a} ≤0.5 cm, T_{1b} >0.5 cm-1 cm, T_{1c} >1 cm-2 cm)
T_2	>2cm-5 cm
T_3	>5 cm
T_{4a}	Involvement of chest wall
T_{4b}	Involvement of skin (includes ulceration, direct infiltration, peau d'orange, and satellite nodules)
T_{4c}	T_{4a} and T_{4b} together
T_{4d}	Inflammatory cancer
N_0	No regional node metastases
N_1	Palpable mobile involved ipsilateral axillary nodes
N_2	Fixed involved ipsilateral axillary nodes
N_3	Ipsilateral internal mammary node involvement (rarely clinically detectable)
M_0	No evidence of metastasis
M_1	Distant metastasis (includes ipsilateral supraclavicular nodes)

Correlation of UICC (1987) and TNM classifications of tumours

UICC stage	TNM classification
I	T_1, N_0, M_0
II	T_1, N_1, M_0; T_2, N_{0-1}, M_0
III	any T, N_{2-3}, M_0; T_3, any N, M_0; T_4, any N, M_0
IV	any T, any N, M_1

When an invasive breast cancer is diagnosed the extent of the disease should be assessed and the tumour staged. The two staging classifications in current use are not well suited to breast cancer: the tumour node metastases (TNM) system depends on clinical measurements and clinical assessment of lymph node status, both of which are inaccurate, and the International Union Against Cancer (UICC) system incorporates the TNM classification. To improve the TNM system, a separate pathological classification has been added; this allows tumour size and node status, as assessed by a pathologist, to be taken into account. Prognosis in breast cancer relates to the stage of the disease at presentation.

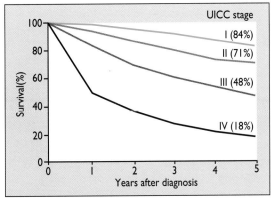

Survival associated with invasive breast cancer according to stage of disease.

To ensure that there is no gross evidence of disease all patients with invasive breast cancer should have a full blood count, liver function tests, and a chest radiograph. Patients with stage I and stage II disease have a low incidence of detectable metastatic disease, and in the absence of abnormal results of liver function tests or specific signs or symptoms they should not undergo further investigations to assess metastatic disease. Patients with bigger or more advanced tumours should be considered for bone and liver scans if these could lead to a change in clinical management.

Surgical treatment of localised breast cancer

Most patients will have a combination of local treatments to control local disease and systemic treatment for any micrometastatic disease. Local treatments consist of surgery and radiotherapy. Surgery can be an excision of the tumour with surrounding normal breast tissue (breast conservation surgery) or a mastectomy.

Certain clinical and pathological factors may influence selection for breast conservation or mastectomy because of their impact on local recurrence after breast conserving therapy. These include an incomplete initial excision, young age, the presence of an extensive in situ component, the presence of lymphatic or vascular invasion, and histological grade. Young patients are more likely to develop local recurrence than older patients, but this is probably because young patients are more likely to have tumours that have an extensive in situ component, have lymphatic or vascular invasion, and are of high grade.

Risk factors for local recurrence of cancer after breast conservation

Factor	Relative risk
Involved margins	×3
Extensive in situ component	×3
Patient's age <35 (v age >50)	×3
Lymphatic or vascular invasion	×2
Histological grade II or III (v grade I)	×2

Relation between age and local recurrence of cancer after breast conservation

Age (years)	Local recurrence after five years
<35	17%
35-50	12%
>50	6%

Breast cancers suitable for treatment by breast conservation

- Single clinical and mammographic lesion
- Tumour ≤4 cm in diameter
- No sign of local advancement (T_1, T_2 <4 cm), extensive nodal involvement (N_0, N_1), or metastases (M_0)
- Tumour >4 cm in large breast

Patients who are best treated by mastectomy

- Those who prefer treatment by mastectomy
- Those for whom breast conservation treatment would produce an unacceptable cosmetic result (includes most central lesions and carcinomas >4 cm in diameter, although breast conserving surgery is now possible if these lesions are successfully treated by primary systemic therapy)
- Those with either clinical or mammographic evidence of more than one focus of cancer in the breast

Factors associated with increased rates of local recurrence after mastectomy

- Axillary lymph node involvement
- Lymphatic or vascular invasion by cancer
- Grade III carcinoma
- Tumour >4 cm in diameter (pathological)

Follow up schedule after surgery for breast cancer

Breast conservation surgery
Review every six months

Mastectomy
Review every six months for first two years and annually thereafter

Breast conservation surgery

Breast conservation surgery may consist of excision of the tumour with a 1 cm margin of normal tissue (wide local excision) or a more extensive excision of a whole quadrant of the breast (quadrantectomy). The wider the excision the lower the recurrence rate but the worse the cosmetic result. There is no size limit for breast conservation surgery, but adequate excision of lesions over 4 cm produces a poor cosmetic result in most women; thus breast conserving surgery tends to be limited to lesions of 4 cm or less. There is no age limit for breast conservation.

Factors affecting cosmetic outcome—Wider excisions give poorer cosmetic results, and excision of any skin overlying the cancer also affects the cosmetic result. For this reason only dimpled or retracted skin overlying a localised breast cancer should be excised. Operations performed in specialist breast units seem to have better cosmetic results than those performed in non-specialist units. Other factors that influence cosmetic outcome include clearance of axillary nodes and delivery of a radiotherapy boost to the tumour bed.

Mastectomy

About a third of localised breast cancers are unsuitable for treatment by breast conservation but can be treated by mastectomy, and some patients who are suitable for breast conservation surgery opt for mastectomy. Mastectomy removes the breast tissue with some overlying skin, usually including the nipple. The breast is removed from the chest wall muscles (pectoralis major, rectus abdominus, and serratus anterior), which are left intact. Mastectomy should be combined with some form of axillary surgery.

Common complications after mastectomy include formation of seroma, infection, and flap necrosis. Collection of fluid under mastectomy flaps after suction drains have been removed (seroma) occurs in a third to a half of all patients. It is more common after a mastectomy and axillary node clearance than after mastectomy and node sampling. The seroma can be aspirated if it is troublesome. Infection after mastectomy is uncommon, and when it occurs it is usually secondary to flap necrosis. Occasionally areas of necrotic skin need to be excised and skin grafts applied. Most patients treated by mastectomy are suitable for some form of breast reconstruction, which should ideally be performed at the same time as the initial mastectomy.

Follow up of patients after surgery

Local recurrence after mastectomy is most common in the first two years and decreases with time. In contrast local recurrence after breast conservation occurs at a fixed rate each year. Follow up schedules should take this difference into account. The aim of follow up is to detect local recurrence while it is treatable or to detect contralateral disease. Patients with carcinoma of one breast are at high risk of cancer in the other breast, and about 1% a year develop this. All patients under follow up after breast cancer should, therefore, have mammography performed regularly (the interval between mammograms varies from one to two years in different units) on one or both breasts. Mammograms can be difficult to interpret after breast conservation because scarring from surgery can result in the formation of a stellate opacity and localised distortion, which can be difficult to differentiate from cancer recurrence. Magnetic resonance imaging seems to be useful in this situation.

Radiotherapy

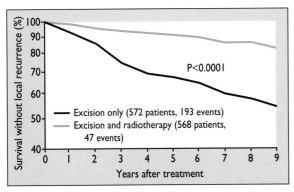

Effect of radiotherapy on local recurrence after wide local excision.

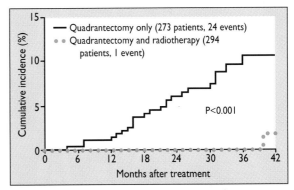

Effect of radiotherapy on local recurrence after quadrantectomy.

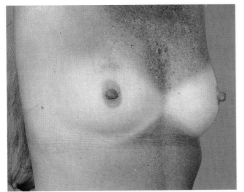

Good cosmetic result after breast conserving surgery and breast radiotherapy.

Studies have shown that all patients should receive radiotherapy to the breast after wide local excision or quadrantectomy. Doses of 40-50 Gy are delivered in daily fractions over three to five weeks. A top up or boost of 15-20 Gy can be given to the excision site either by external beam irradiation or by means of radioactive implants, although it is not yet clear whether a boost is necessary. After mastectomy radiotherapy is only required for patients at high risk of local recurrence: patients with involvement of pectoralis major or any two of the other factors associated with increased risk should be given postoperative radiotherapy.

Complications

With modern machinery and the delivery of smaller fractions the dose of radiotherapy delivered to the skin is minimised. This has dramatically reduced the incidence of immediate skin reactions and subsequent skin telangiectasia. With tangential fields, only a part of the left anterior descending artery and a small fraction of lung tissue are now routinely included within radiotherapy fields, and the risks of cardiac damage and of pneumonitis are low. Reports of increased cardiac deaths many years after radiotherapy for left sided breast cancer relate to old radiotherapy techniques which delivered higher doses of radiotherapy to a much greater proportion of the heart.

Radiation pneumonitis, which is usually transient, affects less than 2% of patients treated with tangential fields. Rib doses are also smaller, with the consequence that rib damage is now much less common than it used to be. In the past there were problems with overlapping radiotherapy fields, resulting in an increased dose of radiation to a small area. If this occurs in the axilla it can cause brachial plexopathy.

Cutaneous radionecrosis and osteoradionecrosis are now rarely seen but do occur in patients who were treated several years ago. Excision of affected areas and reconstruction with local or distant myocutaneous flaps are sometimes necessary as regular antibiotics and dressings rarely result in wound healing.

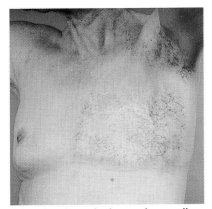

Skin telangiectasia due to chest wall and axillary radiotherapy after mastectomy. This is now rarely seen with modern radiotherapy techniques.

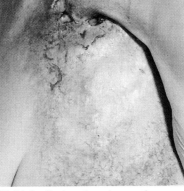

Multiple discharging sinuses from chronic osteomyelitis resulting from rib necrosis due to radiotherapy after radical mastectomy 30 years before.

The sources of the data presented in graphs are: C W Elston and I O Ellis, *Histopathology* 1992;**19**:403-10 for survival associated with tumour grade; B Fisher and C Redmond, *Monogr Natl Cancer Inst* 1992;**11**:7-13 for recurrence after wide local excision; and U Veronesi *et al*, *N Engl J Med* 1993;**328**:1587-91 (copyright Massachusetts Medical Society) for recurrence after quadrantectomy. The data are reproduced with permission of the journals or copyright holders.

MANAGEMENT OF REGIONAL NODES IN BREAST CANCER

N J Bundred, D A L Morgan, J M Dixon

Lymph drainage of breast

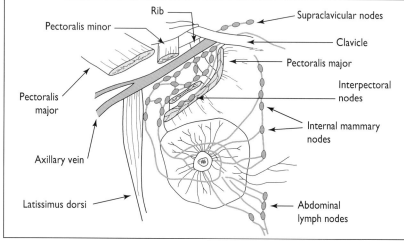

Lymph drainage of breast.

Lymph drainage from the breast is important in relation to malignant disease and is via the axillary and internal mammary nodes. To a lesser extent lymph also drains by intercostal routes to nodes adjacent to the vertebra. The axillary nodes receive about three quarters of the total lymph drainage, and this is reflected in the greater frequency of tumour metastases to these nodes.

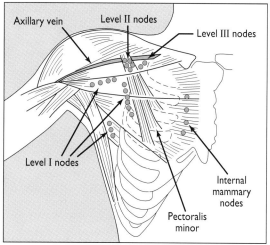

Levels of axillary nodes.

The axillary nodes, which lie below the axillary vein, can be divided into three groups in relation to the pectoralis minor muscle: level I nodes lie lateral to the muscle; level II (central) nodes lie behind the muscle; and level III (apical) nodes lie between the muscle's medial border, the first rib, and the axillary vein. There are on average 20 nodes in the axilla, with about 13 nodes at level I, five at level II, and two at level III. The drainage from level I nodes passes into the central nodes and on into the apical nodes. An alternative route, by which lymph can get to level III nodes without passing through nodes at level I, is through lymph nodes on the undersurface of the pectoralis major muscle, the interpectoral nodes. The orderly drainage of lymph explains why very few patients with cancer have lymph nodes involved at levels II or level III without involvement at level I. These so called skip metastases are seen in less than 5% of patients with axillary node involvement.

Factors affecting lymph node involvement

Factors associated with lymph node involvement

- Large tumour
- Poorly differentiated tumour (grade III)
- Symptomatic (compared with screen detected) tumour
- Presence of lymphatic or vascular invasion in and around tumour
- Oestrogen receptor negative tumour

Preoperative clinical or radiological assessment of lymph node involvement is inaccurate, with only 70% of involved nodes being clinically detectable. Only histopathological assessment of excised nodes provides accurate prognostic information.

Lymph nodes are ineffective barriers to the spread of cancer, and metastasis indicates biologically aggressive disease that requires systemic adjuvant treatment. Involvement of axillary nodes occurs in up to half of symptomatic breast cancers and in 10-20% of screen detected breast cancers.

Role of axillary surgery in patients with operable breast cancer

---

Options for axillary surgery

Procedures to stage but not treat the axilla
- Axillary node sampling (removal of at least four lymph nodes)
- Partial axillary dissection (level I or level I and II)

Procedures to stage and treat the axilla
- Level III dissection

Axillary surgery can be used to stage the axilla or to treat axillary disease, or both.

Staging the axilla

The presence or absence of involved axillary lymph nodes is the single best predictor of survival of breast cancer, and important treatment decisions are based on it. Both the number of involved nodes and the level of nodal involvement predict survival from breast cancer. Only nodal involvement that is evident on routine histopathological examination is of proved prognostic importance. The prognostic value of finding microscopic metastases in lymph nodes either by examining multiple sections or by immunohistochemistry remains to be determined.

A single node biopsy does not adequately stage the axilla. Although some centres have found that sampling (dissecting out four separate nodes) provides reliable information on whether axillary nodes are involved, others have found it difficult to identify and dissect out four separate axillary nodes. The probability of a false negative result on sampling decreases as the number of nodes sampled increases. A level I dissection, which should contain at least 10 nodes, provides information on whether there are axillary nodal metastases but does not provide definitive evidence of the number of involved axillary nodes. Level II or III dissections (removing all nodes at levels I and II or I, II, and III) provide more accurate assessments of the number and level of node involvement.

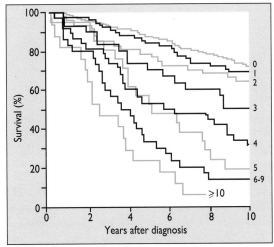

Relation between number of involved axillary lymph nodes and survival after breast cancer.

Treatment of axillary disease

A partial (level I or level II) dissection or sampling of axillary nodes cannot be considered as treatments because even if there is only a single node metastasis at level I there is a 12·5% chance of nodes at level II or III being involved, and if there is metastasis at level II there is a 50% incidence of level III nodal involvement. Thus, patients who are found by axillary sampling or level I and II dissections to have involved axillary nodes require radical axillary radiotherapy; patients with negative nodes after these axillary staging procedures require no further treatment to the axilla.

Some surgeons deliberately limit their axillary dissection to level II, arguing that this carries a lower incidence of complications than a level III dissection and that patients with nodal involvement at level II will receive adjuvant systemic treatment that will control residual apical nodal disease. Both assumptions are unproved, and residual disease at the apex of the axilla can cause distressing symptoms that can be difficult to treat. Although axillary radiotherapy given after a level II dissection will control metastases at level III, this combination of procedures is associated with high rates of lymphoedema (>30%).

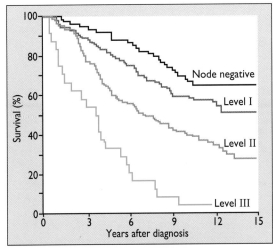

Relation between level of axillary lymph node involvement and survival after breast cancer.

Control of axillary disease

Axillary recurrence in 10 years after level III axillary clearance, radiotherapy, or watch policy*

	Clearance	Radiotherapy	Watch policy
Axillary relapse	3%	8%	21%
Uncontrolled axillary relapse	1%	5%	12%

*Data compiled from reports from several centres relating to series of symptomatic patients, of whom about half had histologically positive nodes. No patients received adjuvant systemic therapy, which reduces rate of regional node relapse.

The options for treating involved axillary nodes are radical radiotherapy or a level III axillary clearance. Both options provide satisfactory rates of disease control, but a level III axillary clearance seems to provide a lower rate of axillary recurrence. Radiotherapy to the axilla cannot be repeated.

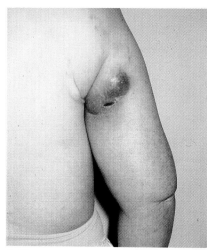

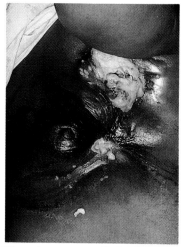

Axillary recurrence causing lymphoedema.

Ulcerating, uncontrolled axillary recurrence.

Some clinicians believe that surgeons should not enter the axilla and that patients should have either radical radiotherapy or a watch policy—treatment of only those patients who develop symptomatic axillary relapse. A watch policy, however, prevents the acquisition of important information that is used both to decide adjuvant treatment and to discuss prognosis with the patient. Uncontrolled axillary recurrence, which can manifest as ulceration or brachial neuropathy, is unpleasant and difficult to treat and is seen more commonly after a watch policy than after an axillary node clearance or radical axillary radiotherapy. The aim of treating the axilla is to minimise axillary relapse; it is evident that such treatment almost certainly has no effect on overall survival.

Morbidity of axillary treatments

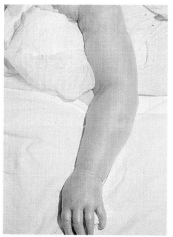

Lymphoedema due to recurrent axillary disease.

Damage to nerves in the axilla may occur during surgery, the most common being division of the sensory intercostobrachial nerve. Many surgeons take care to preserve the intercostobrachial nerve during axillary node surgery, which reduces the number of patients who develop numbness and paraesthesiae down the upper inner aspect of the arm. Radiotherapy may result in brachial plexopathy. This complication may be due in part to overlap of fields, which can result in high doses of radiation being delivered to the brachial plexus. With modern planning techniques, treatment schedules, and newer equipment this complication is rare. Brachial plexopathy can also be due to apical axillary recurrence; this complication is much less common if initial treatment of axillary disease has been optimal.

Wound infection complicates about 5% of axillary surgical procedures and is more common after axillary clearance than sampling: about one third of patients develop seromas after a level III axillary clearance compared with less than 5% of patients who undergo four node sampling.

Reduced range of movement—Both surgery and radiotherapy are associated with a reduction in the range of movement of the shoulder in some patients, and about 5% develop a frozen shoulder. This can be minimised with regular exercise programmes developed and supervised by physiotherapists, and patients with a frozen shoulder require a prolonged course of intensive physiotherapy.

Methods for control of lymphoedema

- Oral bioflavonoid oxerutins or coumarin
- Bandaging arm
- Elasticated compression sleeve (should be individually measured for each patient)
- Multiple chamber Flowtron pumps (must be used for at least two hours a day to maintain improvement)

Symptomatic lymphoedema occurs in less than 5% of patients treated by a level II or III axillary dissection or by radical radiotherapy. It is much more common when an extensive axillary dissection (such as a level II dissection) is combined with radical radiotherapy. Radiotherapy should not be given after a level III axillary dissection. Recurrence in the axilla produces the most extreme lymphoedema. There is no satisfactory treatment for this problem, but symptoms can be improved and, in some patients, the lymphoedema controlled.

Treatment of internal mammary and supraclavicular nodes

The value of prophylactic irradiation of the internal mammary and supraclavicular nodal areas is unproved. For anatomical and geometric reasons the supraclavicular nodes can readily be included when axillary radiotherapy is given and, providing there is no overlap of fields, adds little in the way of morbidity. Such treatment reduces the rate of supraclavicular recurrence but has no impact on survival.

Over 90% of women with metastases to the internal mammary nodes have axillary node involvement. Of the 5-10% who have internal mammary node involvement in isolation, most have tumours involving the medial half of the breast. Some surgeons take biopsy samples from the internal mammary chain (through the second intercostal space) of patients aged under 60 who have medial tumours. Such patients are candidates for systemic chemotherapy if they are node positive.

Internal mammary nodes can be irradiated only by means of complex fields that include the heart and are no longer routinely covered in radiotherapy fields after mastectomy or wide local excision.

Recommended management of axillary nodes

Recommended management of axillary nodes in patients with operable invasive breast cancer

Premenopausal women

Axillary staging
● Mandatory for all patients

Level III dissection
● Patients with palpable clinically involved nodes
● Patients undergoing mastectomy and reconstruction

Choice of level III dissection or axillary sampling
● All other patients

Postmenopausal women

Level III dissection
● Patients with palpable clinically involved nodes

Choice of level III dissection or axillary sampling
● All other patients with palpable breast cancers

Choice of axillary sampling or watch policy
● Patients with impalpable cancers (<1 cm in diameter)

Premenopausal patients must all have a surgical axillary staging procedure, and a level III axillary dissection has the advantage that it permits identification of patients with a poor outlook—more than 10 nodes positive—who might benefit from more intensive systemic treatment. Removal of nodes at all levels is preferred after mastectomy because it allows all patients to avoid axillary radiotherapy and most to avoid chest wall radiotherapy—this is particularly important for patients who undergo immediate breast reconstruction by tissue expansion.

Postmenopausal women with symptomatic and palpable screen detected cancer should have some form of axillary surgery. As with younger women, full level III axillary clearance is usually preferred after mastectomy. For patients with impalpable tumours (<1 cm in size) the choice is between axillary node sampling (level I dissection or four node sampling) and a watch policy because of the low incidence of axillary node metastases in these patients (<10%). Axillary sampling can be performed at the same time as a therapeutic wide local excision of an impalpable breast cancer that has been diagnosed by image guided fine needle aspiration cytology. If a diagnostic excision of an impalpable breast cancer shows it to have risk factors for nodal involvement the options for treatment are full axillary clearance or axillary sampling.

Presentation of breast cancer with enlarged axillary nodes

Less than 1 in 300 patients with breast cancers present with nodal metastases and an occult primary cancer. Up to 70% of women shown histologically to have metastatic adenocarcinoma in the axillary nodes will have an occult breast cancer, most of which will be visible on mammography. Treament of these 70% is as for breast cancer with palpable nodal metastases. In the remaining 30% axillary node clearance (level I, II, and III dissection) should be performed and the breast kept under regular observation or irradiated. Both groups of patients should receive appropriate adjuvant systemic treatment.

Treatment of axillary recurrence

Treatment depends on whether recurrence occurs in isolation or in association with other sites of recurrence. If initial axillary therapy has been suboptimal, axillary disease can represent residual untreated disease rather than recurrence. Isolated mobile axillary recurrences should be excised and combined with a level III dissection if this has not already been performed. Patients with isolated inoperable recurrence may be given radiotherapy (if not previously given) or systemic treatment, or both; these are sometimes effective at palliation but rarely produce long lasting control of disease. When the disease occurs in association with metastases at other sites systemic treatment is indicated. The most effective strategy is to try to prevent recurrence by ensuring adequate initial treatment.

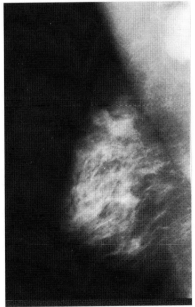

Malignant axillary node visible on mammography with no associated breast lesion.

The picture of axillary recurrence causing lymphoedema has been reproduced from N J Bundred and R E Mansell, eds, *Wolfe coloured atlas of breast disease* (London: Wolfe Medical Publications) 1994 with permission of the publishers.

BREAST CANCER: TREATMENT OF ELDERLY PATIENTS AND UNCOMMON CONDITIONS

J M Dixon, J R C Sainsbury, A Rodger

Treatment of elderly patients

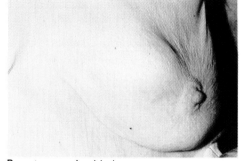

Breast cancer in elderly woman.

About 40% of all breast cancers occur in women aged over 70. The cancers that develop in older women are as aggressive as those seen in younger patients. Treatment with tamoxifen alone controls local disease in less than 30% of elderly patients at five years after diagnosis, which is not satisfactory since the average life expectancy of a 70 year old woman is 14 years. Even when this treatment is restricted to patients with tumours that are oestrogen receptor positive, only half gain long term control of local disease.

Elderly women with breast cancer should be treated in a similar way to younger patients. Few patients are truly unfit for surgery because wide local excision or even mastectomy can, if necessary, be performed under local anaesthesia with sedation. There is no evidence to suggest that elderly patients cannot tolerate radiotherapy as well as younger patients, and when radiotherapy is given it should be given in a radical dose.

Management of elderly patients with breast cancer

Tumour stage and size	Treatment options
T_1 or $T_2 \leqslant 4$ cm size, N_{0-1}, M_0	Wide local excision, node sampling or clearance, and radiotherapy *or* Mastectomy, node clearance, and adjuvant tamoxifen

$T_2 > 4$ cm or T_3, N_{0-1}, M_0:
   Oestrogen receptor:
     Positive
	Mastectomy, node clearance, and adjuvant tamoxifen *or* Tamoxifen and then, if tumour regresses, wide local excision, node sampling or clearance, and radiotherapy

Unknown, negative, or no response to tamoxifen	Mastectomy, node clearance, and adjuvant tamoxifen

T_4, N_2, M_0:
   Oestrogen receptor:
     Positive
	Tamoxifen

Unknown, negative, or no response to tamoxifen	Radical radiotherapy *or in selected patients* Mastectomy and radiotherapy Possibly chemotherapy

Any T, any N, M_1:
   Oestrogen receptor:
     Positive or unknown
	Tamoxifen and symptomatic treatment

Negative	Symptomatic treatment and possibly low dose epirubicin or mitozantrone
Very elderly or infirm patients	Tamoxifen

Operable tumours $\leqslant 4$ cm in size

The alternative treatments are breast conservation surgery (wide local excision, sampling or clearance of axillary nodes, and radiotherapy) or mastectomy and node clearance. Many older women are unhappy about losing a breast and choose breast conservation. Simple mastectomy alone is associated with an unacceptable rate of axillary relapse. Mastectomy and axillary node clearance has a similar postoperative mortality (<1%) to simple mastectomy but is associated with a significantly lower rate of axillary recurrence. Similar mortality is seen after wide local excision, but morbidity is much less after this procedure. All elderly patients, regardless of node status, should be offered adjuvant treatment with tamoxifen.

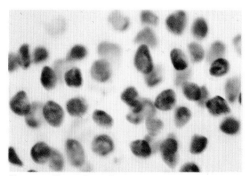

Fine needle aspirate from breast cancer stained for oestrogen receptor: nuclei stained brown indicate cells that are receptor positive.

Operable tumours >4 cm in size

Treatment can be either mastectomy and axillary node clearance or, if the tumour is shown to be oestrogen receptor positive by biopsy or fine needle aspiration cytology, an initial three month course of tamoxifen. During this time the tumour should be monitored: two thirds of women with oestrogen receptor positive tumours will show a regression of their disease to a lower stage after tamoxifen treatment and will become eligible for breast conserving treatment. Patients who have not responded after three months should undergo mastectomy and clearance of axillary nodes. All patients should be given adjuvant tamoxifen.

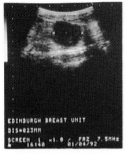
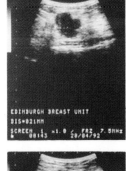

Serial ultrasound scans of breast tumour during three months after tamoxifen treatment: tumour significantly reduced in volume.

Locally advanced breast cancer

In up to a half of patients with oestrogen receptor positive tumours tamoxifen treatment will cause regression of their disease to an extent that some form of local surgery is appropriate. Patients with oestrogen receptor positive tumours that show no response by three months and patients with oestrogen receptor negative tumours should receive adequate locoregional treatment. This is usually radical radiotherapy to the breast, chest wall, and axillary nodes with full dose to skin. Selected patients may alternatively be offered mastectomy or wide local excision with radiotherapy or, occasionally, low dose chemotherapy.

Metastatic disease

Patients with oestrogen receptor positive tumours should receive tamoxifen and appropriate symptomatic treatments. Patients with oestrogen receptor negative tumours should be treated symptomatically. Palliative chemotherapy may provide a worthwhile response without appreciable toxicity in suitable patients.

Very elderly or infirm patients

A small group of very elderly or infirm patients are unfit for treatments other than tamoxifen. These are the only patients for whom tamoxifen should be considered as sole treatment.

Paget's disease of the nipple

Paget's disease of the nipple

- Associated with 1-2% of all breast cancers
- Occurs in similar age range as other breast cancers
- Often associated with delay in diagnosis
- Diagnosis established by cytology or wedge biopsy of nipple

Treatment
- Mass lesion—mastectomy, axillary node clearance, and radiotherapy (or rarely wide local excision, node sampling or clearance, and radiotherapy)
- No mass lesion—wide local excision, node sampling, and radiotherapy or mastectomy and node sampling

---

Paget's disease is an eczematoid change of the nipple associated with an underlying breast malignancy, and about 1-2% of patients with breast cancer have it. In half of these patients it is associated with an underlying mass lesion, and 90% of such patients will have an invasive carcinoma. Of the patients without a mass lesion, 30% will later be found to have an invasive carcinoma and the remainder have in situ disease alone.

Paget's disease may be localised or occupy a large area; the lesion should be differentiated from eczema affecting the nipple and from direct spread into the nipple by an adjacent invasive carcinoma. Clinically, Paget's disease affects the nipple from the start, whereas eczema affects the areolar region first and only rarely affects the nipple skin. If Paget's disease is suspected on clinical examination, mammography should be performed to determine if there is an underlying lesion. Imprint cytology (pressing the eczematoid lesion onto a slide) or scrape cytology (scraping some of the lesion onto a slide) can sometimes establish the diagnosis. The most reliable method of obtaining a diagnosis is by incisional biopsy—removing a portion of the abnormal skin for pathological examination.

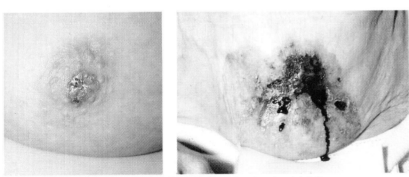

Paget's disease of the nipple: localised (left) and extensive (right).

Management

If a mass lesion is present the appropriate treatment is mastectomy and axillary node clearance (60% of patients with a mass lesion have involved axillary nodes). When Paget's disease is associated with an underlying central lesion a wide excision of the nipple, areola, and underlying mass followed by radiotherapy can give a satisfactory cosmetic result and satisfactory control of local disease. Adjuvant treatment depends on nodal and menopausal status.

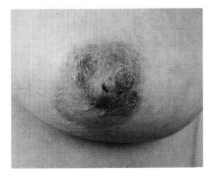
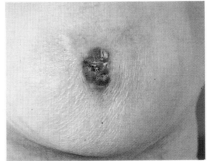

Eczema of the nipple.   *Nipple directly involved by breast cancer.*

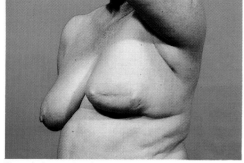

Cosmetic result of treating Paget's disease and underlying mass lesion by wide excision of mass and nipple and areolar complex.

For patients without a mass lesion wide local excision alone is associated with a high rate of local recurrence, but adjuvant radiotherapy may increase rates of local control to acceptable levels. Mastectomy and axillary node sampling (less than 10% of patients without a clinical mass have nodal metastases) is the standard treatment and provides long term disease control in over 95% of patients.

Breast cancer and pregnancy

Breast cancer during pregnancy

- Affects 1-3 of every 10 000 pregnancies
- 25% of all breast cancers in women aged <35 associated with pregnancy
- 15% of all breast cancers in women aged <40 associated with pregnancy
- 65% of pregnant women with breast cancer have involved axillary nodes

Treatment
- First and second trimester—mastectomy and axillary node clearance
- Third trimester—ideally delay treatment and deliver baby at 30-32 weeks; consider primary systemic treatment if tumour large or locally advanced; consider mastectomy, node clearance, and radiotherapy if tumour growing rapidly

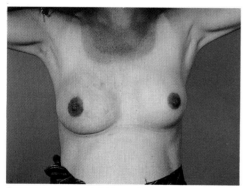

Breast cancer of right breast during pregnancy.

About 1-2% of all breast cancers occur during pregnancy or during lactation, and a quarter of women who develop breast cancer under the age of 35 do so either during or within one year of pregnancy. There is no evidence that breast cancer occurring during pregnancy is more aggressive than other breast cancer, but diagnosis is often delayed because of the difficulty of identifying a discrete mass in an enlarging breast. This means that women tend to present with cancers at a later stage, about 65% having involved axillary nodes.

Management
Treatment during the first two trimesters is a modified radical mastectomy. Radiotherapy should not be delivered during pregnancy. Chemotherapy can be given but is associated with a small risk of fetal damage, particularly in the early stages of pregnancy. Breast cancer in the third trimester can be managed either by immediate surgery or by monitoring the tumour, delivering the baby early at 30-32 weeks, and then instituting treatment after delivery. This allows patients with large or locally advanced breast cancers to have primary systemic treatment, which can sometimes cause regression of the disease to a lower stage at which less extensive surgery can be performed. When monitoring shows the tumour to be increasing in size, treatment (surgery or chemotherapy, depending on which is appropriate) should be instituted before delivery.

Pregnancy after treatment of breast cancer
There is only limited information on the effect of pregnancy on the outcome of a patient with breast cancer. It is generally recommended that there should be a delay of two to three years between treatment for breast cancer and pregnancy because most relapses (80%) occur in the first two years. Women given breast conserving treatment including radiotherapy have on occasions breast fed from the treated breast with no deleterious effects to mother or baby.

Male breast cancer

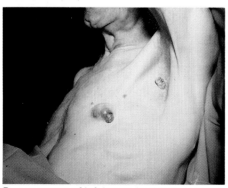

Breast cancer of left breast in elderly man.

Less than 0·5% of all breast cancers occur in men, and breast cancer comprises 0·7% of all male cancers. The peak incidence is five to 10 years later than it is in women. Klinefelter's syndrome is the only known risk factor for male breast cancer.

Presentation is usually with a lump or retraction of the skin or nipple. Male breast cancers are usually eccentric masses whereas gynaecomastia is almost always central. Infiltration of the skin or nipple occurs much earlier in male breast cancer because of the smaller breast volume, and, compared with female breast cancer, the disease is more likely to be advanced at diagnosis. Mammography is valuable in determining whether breast enlargement is due to gynaecomastia or breast cancer. When there is doubt fine needle aspiration should be performed to establish a definitive diagnosis. The histology and prognosis for each tumour stage are similar to those for female breast cancer.

Male breast cancer

- 0·7% of all male cancers
- 0·5% of all breast cancers
- Peak incidence 5-10 years later than in women
- Klinefelter's syndrome increases risk
- Diagnosis by mammography and fine needle aspiration cytology

Treatment
- Mastectomy, axillary node clearance, and radiotherapy
- Adjuvant tamoxifen
- Consider adjuvant chemotherapy in fit patients if tumour oestrogen receptor negative and axillary nodes involved

Management

Treatment of localised breast cancer is usually by modified radical mastectomy (mastectomy and clearance of axillary nodes) and radiotherapy to the chest wall; radiotherapy is given because it is more difficult to get wide excision margins in males and the disease is often locally advanced. Small breast cancers can be treated by wide local excision with sampling or clearance of axillary nodes and postoperative radiotherapy. Adjuvant tamoxifen is effective at reducing recurrence, but adjuvant chemotherapy should be considered for fit patients with tumours that have nodal involvement and that are oestrogen receptor negative. Local recurrence or metastatic disease can be treated by castration (surgical or medical). Systemic chemotherapy should be considered for fit patients with life threatening disease or with symptomatic, recurrent, or metastatic disease that does not respond to castration. The regimens are identical to those used in female breast cancer.

Other rare neoplasms

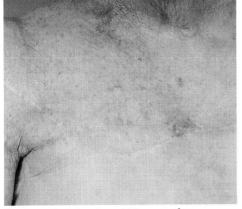

Mammogram showing multiple lymphomatous deposits in breast and regional nodes.

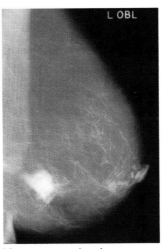

Mammogram showing suspicious abnormality that was subsequently found to be fibromatosis.

Lymphomas rarely occur in the breast: staging investigations are necessary for patients with lymphoma because they usually also have disease outside the regional nodes. Localised lymphoma should be treated by excision, axillary node sampling, radiotherapy, and chemotherapy. The extent of the excision depends on the size of the lesion. Small lesions can be completely excised, but large lesions should be biopsied as they are sensitive to both radiotherapy and chemotherapy. More generalised lymphoma requires systemic chemotherapy.

Proliferative lesions characterised by spindle cells may range from benign overgrowths to sarcomas. Lesions in the middle of this range include fibromatosis and nodular fasciitis, which masquerade clinically and mammographically as breast cancers. They are rare but can recur locally after excision. They should be treated by wide local excision and careful surveillance.

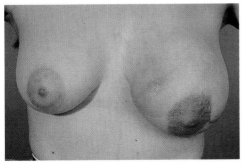

Sarcoma that developed 20 years after radiotherapy to chest wall for breast cancer.

Sarcomas may develop in breast tissue or may affect overlying skin, and, rarely, they may follow radiotherapy to the chest wall. Diagnosis is often suggested by the results of fine needle aspiration cytology. Sarcomas are best treated by as wide an excision as possible; since many of these tumours are large at diagnosis, mastectomy is generally necessary. Axillary node sampling is adequate because axillary nodes are rarely involved. Radiotherapy should be given to the chest wall after excisional surgery, but there is no evidence that adjuvant chemotherapy is of benefit. Survival seems to be related to the size and grade of the tumour.

Phyllodes tumours are rare fibroepithelial neoplasms that range from benign to malignant in their behaviour, though most are benign. Up to 20% recur locally after excision. In the more malignant lesions it is the sarcomatous element that recurs, and almost a quarter of those lesions classified as malignant metastasize. Initial treatment is by wide excision, and mastectomy is often required. The role of radiotherapy and chemotherapy in treating these lesions is unclear.

Recurrent malignant phyllodes tumour in left breast of 19 year old woman. Her initial excision had been two months previously.

ROLE OF SYSTEMIC TREATMENT FOR PRIMARY OPERABLE BREAST CANCER

M A Richards, I E Smith

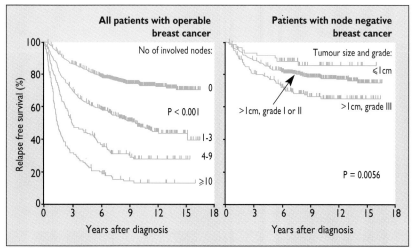

Survival without relapse of patients with operable breast cancer (data from Guy's Hospital, London).

Over half of women with operable breast cancer who receive locoregional treatment alone (surgery with or without radiotherapy) will die from metastatic disease, indicating that for most women the cancer has already spread by the time of presentation. The major risk factors for development of metastases are axillary lymph nodes being involved, an adverse histological grade (indicating an undifferentiated cancer), and large tumour size. Combinations of these factors can be used to define groups with widely different risks of relapse: from less than 10% to more than 90% remaining free of disease after five years. The only way to improve the chance of survival for many of these women is to give them effective systemic treatment.

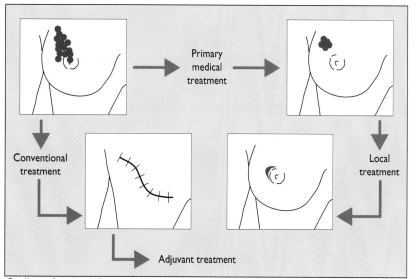

Outline of options for systemic treatment of large, operable breast cancer.

Systemic treatment may be given either as adjuvant treatment after locoregional treatment or as primary systemic treatment before locoregional treatment. The effectiveness of adjuvant treatment has been clearly shown in clinical trials, while primary systemic treatment is still being evaluated. A problem with adjuvant treatment is that its effectiveness in individual patients cannot be assessed as there is no overt disease to monitor. In contrast the effectiveness of primary medical treatment can be assessed by monitoring the size of the primary tumour. Primary medical treatment in operable breast cancer can result in shrinkage of a tumour; thus, a large tumour initially treatable only by mastectomy can be made suitable for breast conserving treatment.

Advantages and disadvantages of adjuvant and primary systemic treatment

Systemic treatment	Advantages	Disadvantages
Adjuvant	Proved efficacy	Uncertainty whether treatment is effective in individual patients
	Prognostic information available after surgery	
Primary	Allows direct assessment of effectiveness	Loss of prognostic information
	Tumour shrinkage may allow breast conservation	May treat in situ disease (if diagnosis made by fine needle aspiration cytology alone)

One potential problem with primary systemic treatment is that, if the diagnosis of cancer is made by fine needle aspiration cytology alone, in situ disease could be treated by chemotherapy (cytology cannot differentiate invasive and in situ disease). For this reason most units perform core or incisional biopsy to obtain a histological diagnosis of invasive cancer before embarking on primary medical treatment. There is no evidence that leaving a primary tumour in the breast during primary systemic treatment increases a patient's anxiety.

Adjuvant treatment

Improvements in 10 year survival of women with stage II breast cancer associated with different treatments*

Treatment	Proportional reduction in annual mortality (SD)	Absolute reduction in 10 year mortality per 100 women treated (SD)
Women aged ≥50		
Polychemotherapy† only	12% (4%)	5 (2)
Tamoxifen only (for median of 2 years)	20% (2%)	8 (1)
Polychemotherapy† and tamoxifen	30% (5%)	12 (2)
Women aged <50		
Polychemotherapy† only	25% (5%)	10 (3)
Ovarian ablation only	28% (9%)	11 (4)
Polychemotherapy† and ovarian ablation‡	30-40%	12-16

*Absolute benefit may be about half as great for stage I cancer.
†For example, 6 months of cyclophosphamide, methotrexate, and fluorouracil.
‡Estimates unreliable because of small amount of data.

Side effects of drugs used for adjuvant treatment

Chemotherapy
- Fatigue and lethargy
- Alopecia (temporary)
- Nausea and vomiting
- Induction of menopause
- Specific side effects of certain drugs
- Risk of infection
- Oral mucositis
- Diarrhoea
- Weight gain

Oophorectomy
- Induction of menopause
- Vaginal dryness
- Hot flushes
- Osteoporosis

Gonadotrophin releasing hormone analogues
- As for oophorectomy
- Pain and bruising at injection site

Tamoxifen
- Hot flushes
- Altered libido
- Gastrointestinal upset
- Visual disturbances—rare (stop drug if reported)
- Vaginal dryness
- Menstrual disturbance
- Weight gain

Antiemetic regimens during chemotherapy

*Moderately emetogenic chemotherapy**
- Intravenous dexamethasone before and after chemotherapy, intravenous metoclopramide, and oral dexamethasone and metoclopramide to take home
- If previous vomiting with chemotherapy or if patient aged <45 consider intravenous ondansetron 8 mg or intravenous granisetron 3 mg before chemotherapy and intravenous dexamethasone 8-16 mg

Highly emetogenic chemotherapy†
- Intravenous ondansetron 8 mg or intravenous granisetron 3 mg, intravenous dexamethasone, and oral dexamethasone to take home

*For example, cyclophosphamide, methotrexate, and fluorouracil.
†Regimens containing high doses of doxorubicin and cisplatin.

Polychemotherapy, oophorectomy, and treatment with tamoxifen produce significant reductions in the annual rates of tumour recurrence and of death. These treatments have been shown to affect survival for at least 10 years and probably longer. The treatments are proportionally as effective for women at high risk of relapse (such as node positive patients) as for women at lower risk, but absolute reduction in mortality is much greater for patients at high risk.

Chemotherapy

From results of clinical trials it is clear that
- A combination of drugs is more effective than a single drug
- A single (perioperative) course of treatment is less effective than a more prolonged course of treatment (six months), but there seems to be no advantage in giving treatment for longer than six months
- The benefits of chemotherapy are greatest in women aged under 50; a smaller but still significant benefit is seen in older women.

Oophorectomy
- Is only of benefit in women aged under 50 (premenopausal)
- Produces survival benefits of similar magnitude to those obtained by polychemotherapy in such younger women
- Can be achieved surgically, by radiation, or by administration of analogues of gonadotrophin releasing hormone.

Tamoxifen
- 20 mg a day is as effective as higher doses
- One year of treatment is less effective than two or more years, and five years may be better than two years
- Reduces the risk of contralateral breast cancer by about 40%
- Benefits are greatest in patients with tumours rich in oestrogen receptors, but smaller reductions in mortality still occur in patients with tumours poor in oestrogen receptors
- Is effective in all age groups

Side effects

Although hair loss is the most common concern of patients before starting chemotherapy, 80% report fatigue and lethargy as the most troublesome side effect. The occurrence of alopecia with some chemotherapy regimens may be reduced by scalp cooling. Nausea and vomiting are unpleasant side effects but can be controlled in most patients by appropriate antiemetic drugs. Younger patients seem to be more at risk of nausea and vomiting and are more likely to suffer from extrapyramidal side effects from standard antiemetic regimens including metoclopramide. It is thus appropriate to give serotonin-3 (5-HT$_3$) antagonists to women aged under 45 as first line treatment even for moderately emetogenic chemotherapy.

The side effects of hormonal treatment are greatest in premenopausal patients. Only 3% of patients given tamoxifen stop taking the drug because of side effects, but vaginal dryness, loss of libido, and hot flushes can have a considerable impact on quality of life. First line treatment for vaginal dryness is with a non-hormonal cream (such as Replens), but if this is not effective creams containing an oestrogen (such as dienoestrol cream) should be tried. Clonidine is occasionally effective at relieving flushing. Evening primrose oil has been reported anecdotally to improve menopausal symptoms, but in controlled trials it has not been shown to be of benefit. Weight gain can be a problem with tamoxifen and with chemotherapy. Tamoxifen has been reported to be associated with an increased incidence of endometrial cancer in postmenopausal women.

Selection of adjuvant treatment

Choice of treatment depends on the risk of relapse, the potential benefit from different forms of treatment, and the acceptability of the treatment to the patient. The risk of relapse relates to known prognostic factors, which can be used to define risk groups. Age or menopausal status is the other important factor that affects choice of adjuvant treatment.

Age

The benefits of adjuvant chemotherapy are considerably greater in women aged under 50 than in older women. There is no satisfactory explanation for this, but it may be partially related to the induction of amenorrhoea after a course of polychemotherapy. Adjuvant chemotherapy is not widely used in women aged over 50 in Britain, but this is not so in the United States. Improvements in survival after ovarian ablation are limited to women aged under 50, but tamoxifen is effective in all age groups.

Which chemotherapy regimen?

Cyclophosphamide, methotrexate, and fluorouracil is the most widely used regimen in the United Kingdom. Whether regimens containing anthracyclines (such as doxorubicin and epirubicin) are superior remains controversial. Some units give regimens containing doxorubicin to premenopausal women at high risk of relapse. Four cycles of doxorubicin and cyclophosphamide seem to be as effective as six cycles of cyclophosphamide, methotrexate, and fluorouracil.

Combinations of chemotherapy and hormonal treatment

For women aged over 50 the effects of tamoxifen and chemotherapy seem to be additive. Tamoxifen, however, has a considerably greater effect on mortality than does chemotherapy in these older, postmenopausal women and less toxicity. Whether the additional benefit justifies the use of chemotherapy in these patients is a matter for individual judgment by both patient and doctor. The effects of combining chemotherapy and hormonal treatment in women aged under 50 are unclear. In many centres patients are entered into trials of adjuvant treatment, which may therefore not follow that outlined here.

Patients at very high risk

Protocols of intensive treatment are being assessed in patients at very high risk. Women with 10 or more positive axillary lymph nodes are being offered high dose chemotherapy with autologous transplantation of bone marrow or harvesting and subsequent rescue of peripheral stem cells. Early results show mortality related to treatment is controllable (less than 5%), but morbidity is high. Comparison with historical controls suggests a prolongation in time to relapse, and preliminary evidence indicates a survival benefit. Randomised controlled clinical trials are currently under way, and results from these studies are required before this treatment is introduced in all units.

Definitions of risk groups and associated risk of relapse

Risk group	Definition	Survival without relapse after 5 years
Node negative patients		
• Low risk	Tumour ≤1 cm in diameter	>90%
• Intermediate risk	Tumour >1 cm, grade I or II	75-80%
• High risk	Tumour >1 cm, grade III	50-60%
Node positive patients		
• Low and intermediate risk	1-3 axillary nodes involved	40-50%
• High risk	4-9 axillary nodes involved	20-30%
• Very high risk	≥10 axillary nodes involved	10-15%

Common adjuvant chemotherapy regimens

- Cyclophosphamide, methotrexate, and fluorouracil; repeated every 21-28 days
- Doxorubicin and cyclophosphamide; repeated every 21 days (fluorouracil may be added to regimen, and epirubicin may be substituted for doxorubicin)

Adjuvant treatment for patients with breast cancer

Risk group	Premenopausal patients	Postmenopausal patients
Node negative patients		
• Low risk	Tamoxifen or no treatment	Tamoxifen or no treatment
• Intermediate risk	Tamoxifen	Tamoxifen
• High risk	Consider chemotherapy* (with or without tamoxifen) or Ovarian ablation (with or without tamoxifen) if tumour is oestrogen receptor positive	Tamoxifen (with or without chemotherapy)
Node positive patients		
• Low and intermediate risk	Chemotherapy* (with or without tamoxifen) or Ovarian ablation (with or without tamoxifen) if tumour is oestrogen receptor positive or Chemotherapy* and ovarian ablation (with or without tamoxifen)	Tamoxifen with or without chemotherapy
• High and very high risk	Consider more intensive chemotherapy† (with or without tamoxifen)	Tamoxifen and chemotherapy if fit

*For example, cyclophosphamide, methotrexate, and fluorouracil.
†For example, regimen containing anthracycline. Some units are investigating use of intensive chemotherapy supported by rescue of bone marrow or peripheral stem cells for patients at very high risk.

Primary medical treatment

The use of primary medical (neoadjuvant) treatment for operable breast cancer has increased over the past five years. The main advantages to this approach have already been outlined. Accurate assessment of response is important to determine whether the systemic treatment is effective. Clinical response is assessed according to criteria of the International Union Against Cancer (UICC); mammographic or ultrasonographic assessments of response may also be useful. Both the primary tumour and lymph node metastases can be shown to respond, and invasive cancer seems to be more sensitive to chemotherapy than in situ disease.

Chemotherapy

With conventional regimens for primary systemic chemotherapy, about 70% of patients show a partial response (primary cancer shrinking by >50%), 20-30% show a complete clinical response, and a small number (about 10-15%) achieve a complete pathological response. The regimens used for primary chemotherapy have generally been the same as those used for adjuvant treatment. There is preliminary evidence that continuous infusional chemotherapy with agents such as fluorouracil combined with intermittent agents such as epirubicin and cisplatin achieves higher response rates (over 90%) than bolus chemotherapy.

Hormonal treatments

Tamoxifen (20 mg a day by mouth) produces a partial response in 75% of elderly patients with hormone responsive (oestrogen receptor positive) tumours and a complete clinical response in 15%. The use of gonadotrophin releasing hormone analogues (goserelin 3·6 mg monthly given subcutaneously or leuprorelin 3·75 mg monthly given subcutaneously or intramuscularly) as primary medical treatment for premenopausal women with oestrogen receptor positive tumours is under evaluation in some centres. Few patients show complete pathological responses after hormonal treatment, but the side effects are generally much less than with chemotherapy.

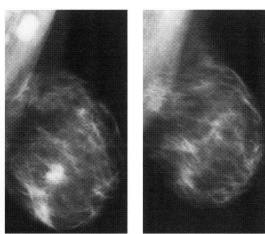

Mammograms of breast showing primary cancer and involved axillary node (left) and after primary chemotherapy (right). At subsequent surgery patient was found to have no residual carcinoma in breast or axilla—complete pathological response.

Outcome

Tumours will show either a useful response or progression within 12 weeks of primary medical treatment. To ensure that women with progressive disease are detected as early as possible, clinical and ultrasonographic assessment of tumour volume should be performed at monthly intervals.

Between 50% and 70% of patients with large tumours will have sufficient tumour regression to avoid mastectomy. All patients require some form of local treatment (surgery or radiotherapy) after primary systemic treatment. It is not yet clear whether primary medical treatment prolongs survival, and a series of randomised trials are under way to assess this.

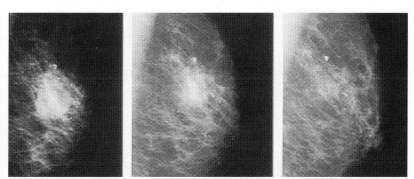

Serial mammograms during primary treatment with systemic chemotherapy. Mass lesion disappeared, but microcalcification remained; subsequent mastectomy showed that the microcalcification was associated with residual carcinoma in situ.

Selection of patients

Primary systemic treatment was initially given to patients with locally advanced (inoperable) breast cancers, and its use has now been extended to patients with large operable breast cancers in an attempt to avoid mastectomy. The use of primary systemic treatment for other groups of patients cannot be recommended (except in clinical trials) until results are available from trials comparing it with standard treatments.

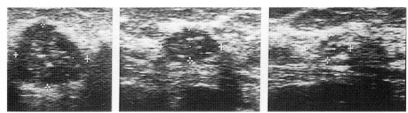

Serial ultrasound scans at fortnightly intervals during primary treatment with chemotherapy.

The data presented in the box of improvements in survival associated with different treatments are from Early Breast Cancer Trialists' Collaborative Group, *Lancet* 1992;**339**:71-85 and are reproduced with permission of the journal.

LOCALLY ADVANCED BREAST CANCER

A Rodger, R C F Leonard, J M Dixon

Clinical features of locally advanced breast cancer

Skin
- Ulceration
- Satellite nodules
- Dermal infiltration
- Peau d'orange
- Erythema over tumour

Chest wall
Tumour fixation to
- Ribs
- Intercostal muscles
- Serratus anterior

Axillary nodes
- Nodes fixed to one another or to other structures

Locally advanced disease of the breast is characterised clinically by features suggesting infiltration of the skin or chest wall by tumour or matted involved axillary nodes. Large operable breast cancers and tumours fixed to muscle should not be considered as locally advanced. Depending on referral patterns and clinical definitions, between one in 12 and one in four patients with breast cancer present with locally advanced disease. Reflecting the differences in definition and the variable natural history of breast cancer, reported five year survival varies between 1% and 30%. Median survival is about 2-2·5 years, which is similar to that described for breast cancer in the late 19th and early 20th centuries.

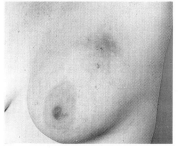

Inflammatory breast carcinoma.

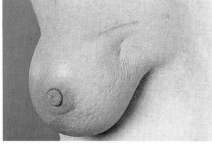

Peau d'orange associated with breast carcinoma.

Locally advanced breast cancer may arise because of its position in the breast (for example, peripheral), neglect (some patients do not present to hospital for month or years after they notice a mass), or biological aggressiveness (this includes all inflammatory cancers and most with peau d'orange). Inflammatory carcinomas are uncommon and are characterised by brawny, oedematous, indurated, and erythematous skin changes and have the worst prognosis of all locally advanced breast cancers.

Treatment

Current treatments have had some impact on control of local disease but have had little overall effect on metastatic progression, although survival is better with hormone sensitive disease. Local and regional relapse is a major problem and affects more than half of patients.

Factors affecting choice of systemic treatment for locally advanced breast cancer

Hormonal treatment
- Slow growing or indolent disease
- Oestrogen receptor positive cancer
- Elderly or unfit patients

Chemotherapy
- Inflammatory cancer
- Oestrogen receptor negative cancer
- Rapidly progressive cancer

Role of systemic and local treatment

The mainstay of local treatment has been radiotherapy. This is because surgery, generally mastectomy, results in high rates of local recurrence. In contrast, radiotherapy alone can produce high rates of local remission in both the breast and axilla, but with radiotherapy alone only 30% of patients remain free of locoregional disease at death. A combination of appropriate systemic treatment and radiotherapy can increase the initial rate of local response to over 80%.

Choice of systemic treatment

Systemic treatment should be administered as part of a planned programme of combined systemic and local treatment. For frail patients treatment may initially be by tamoxifen, with radiotherapy held in reserve for relapse.

Choice of systemic treatment for locally advanced breast cancer

Hormonal treatment
- Premenopausal women—ovarian ablation (surgery, radiation, or gonadotrophin releasing hormone antagonists)
- Postmenopausal women—tamoxifen

Chemotherapy
- Intravenous—infusion of fluorouracil combined with an anthracycline*
- Intra-arterial

*For example, doxorubicin, cyclophosphamide, and fluorouracil; or epirubicin, cisplatin, and fluorouracil.

Although standard chemotherapy regimens have increased rates of local control, they have had little impact on survival. Studies are currently under way to determine whether intensifying drug dosage (increasing the amount of drug given in a fixed period either by giving smaller doses more frequently or by combining higher doses with factors to encourage regeneration of bone marrow) does produce survival benefits. Current data suggest that infusional treatment with fluorouracil combined with the anthracyclines doxorubicin or epirubicin in regimens with cyclophosphamide or cisplatin may produce higher response rates than intermittent regimens used for adjuvant chemotherapy.

Radiotherapy for locally advanced breast cancer

Treatment areas
- Breast
- Axilla and supraclavicular fossa

Treatment
- Megavoltage *x* rays
- Technique for enhancing skin dose
- 40-50 Gy in 15-25 fractions over 3-5 weeks
- Boost to tumour mass if possible by external beam or radioactive implant of 10-20 Gy

Toxicity
- Lethargy
- Skin erythema and small areas of moist desquamation
- Temporary mild dysphagia
- <3% risk of pneumonitis

Radiotherapy

Radiotherapy is generally well tolerated, even by elderly and frail patients. It can be given concurrently with systemic hormonal treatment, or it can be given after a course of primary chemotherapy to patients whose breast cancer still shows signs of local advancement. The breast skin requires full dose, and this will result in temporary erythema and possible desquamation. If possible palpable tumour masses should receive treatment boosts.

Surgery

Mastectomy is generally not indicated in the presence of features of locally advanced disease, but the role of surgery is changing. Intensive treatment with a combination of cytotoxic drugs or initial hormonal treatment often causes the primary tumour to regress to a lower stage (with disappearance of peau d'orange and erythema and reduction in tumour volume), making surgery feasible some weeks or months after the start of systemic treatment. In such cases surgery may be a wide excision and clearance of axillary nodes or a total mastectomy and node clearance, both being followed by radiotherapy to the remaining breast or to the chest wall.

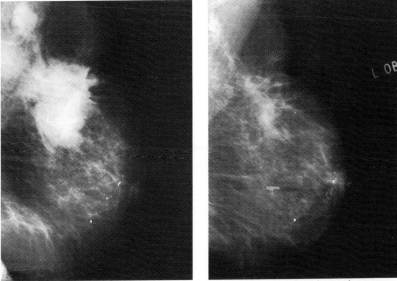

Mammogram of locally advanced breast tumour (left); and after chemotherapy, showing substantial reduction in tumour volume (right). (Tumour was operable after treatment.)

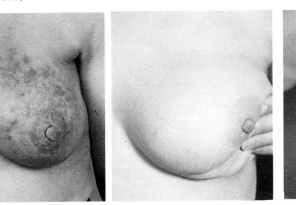

Locally advanced breast cancer (left); and complete clinical response after chemotherapy (right).

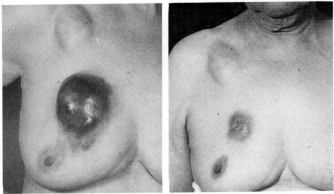

Locally advanced breast cancer (left); and reduction in size after six months of tamoxifen treatment (right). The mass in the infraclavicular region is a lipoma.

Locally advanced breast cancer

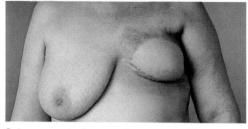

Salvage mastectomy and coverage with myocutaneous flap (from latissimus dorsi) for treatment of residual disease after chemotherapy and radiotherapy.

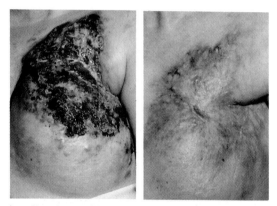

Locally advanced breast cancer with ulceration (left); and good response and re-epithelialisation after three courses of intra-arterial chemotherapy (right).

In some patients residual disease remains in the breast despite systemic treatment and radiotherapy. This disease can be excised by a salvage mastectomy, ideally followed by coverage with a myocutaneous flap (latissimus dorsi or transverse rectus abdominus). "Toilet" surgery, used in an effort to control fungating cancers or recurrence and progression of disease, is often ineffective and should only be performed for breast cancers that are locally advanced either because of their peripheral position in the breast or because of a delay in presentation. In this group surgery should be combined with radiotherapy and appropriate adjuvant systemic treatment.

Intra-arterial chemotherapy

Despite the best efforts with combined treatments, a substantial proportion of patients who present with locally advanced disease develop uncontrolled disease of the chest wall. Although low dose intravenous chemotherapy by infusion (for example, infusional fluorouracil) can relieve symptoms in up to half of these patients, the overall efficacy of systemic chemotherapy is poor. Because of technical difficulties, investigation of intra-arterial chemotherapy has been limited to uncontrolled studies in a few centres. However, the best published series report impressive response rates with low toxicity in patients presenting initially with locally advanced breast cancer. If intra-arterial treatment does not produce a response after the first course it is probably not worth pursuing. The drugs and doses used are similar to those given intravenously for palliative treatment. One problem with delivery of drugs by the intra-arterial route is that in patients who have received radiotherapy the blood vessels supplying the chest wall may be damaged, resulting in an impaired blood supply that limits drug delivery.

Local recurrence after mastectomy

Treatment of local recurrence in chest wall

Type of recurrence	Treatment
Single spot	Excise and consider radiotherapy
Multiple spot	Radiotherapy unless already given or more radical excision (possibly with coverage with myocutaneous flap)
Widespread	Consider radiotherapy unless already given or disease too widespread Appropriate systemic treatment (hormonal or chemotherapy) Intra-arterial chemotherapy Intravenous infusion of fluorouracil

This usually occurs in the skin flaps adjacent to the scar and is presumed to arise from viable cells shed during surgery. It can usually be diagnosed by fine needle aspiration cytology. Local disease can be isolated, but in up to half of patients it heralds systemic relapse. For this reason a search for distant metastases should be undertaken in all patients.

Local recurrence after mastectomy can be classified as single spot relapse, multiple spot relapse, or field change. Treatment and prognosis differ for these three categories.

Treatment

If the recurrence is focal and occurs many years after the original surgery excision alone can provide long term control. If the recurrence is not single but still localised then the options are radiotherapy or a more radical excision. In a more widespread recurrence standard treatments are often disappointing, although intra-arterial chemotherapy and infusional fluorouracil are sometimes effective. Failure to halt the progress of local disease can lead to cancer en cuirasse—where the chest wall is encircled by tumour—a most unpleasant situation for the patient.

Recurrence on the chest wall can be quite indolent, grow slowly, and occur in the absence of metastases elsewhere. The control of ulceration and focal malodorous infected tissue is a considerable problem for carers, and patients with such disease have a miserable existence. Excision of dead tissue and the use of topical and oral antibiotics with antianaerobic activity combined with charcoal dressings help to control the malodour. The best form of treatment is prevention by ensuring that initial local treatment is optimal.

Longstanding, isolated, large, unsightly, and malodorous local recurrence after mastectomy and radiotherapy.

Photographs of the patient treated by intra-arterial chemotherapy were provided by Mr J R C Sainsbury, consultant surgeon at Huddersfield Royal Infirmary.

METASTATIC BREAST CANCER

R C F Leonard, A Rodger, J M Dixon

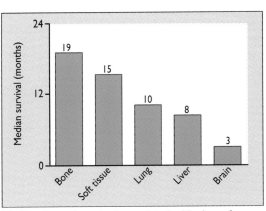

Median time of survival associated with sites of metastasis in patients with breast cancer.

Few other cancers when they metastasise have such a variable natural course and effect on survival as breast cancer. Patients with hormone sensitive cancers may live for several years without any intervention other than various sequential hormonal manipulations. In contrast, patients with disease that is not hormone sensitive have a much shorter interval free of disease and shorter survival, reflecting the more aggressive biology of hormone independent cancers. The average period of survival after diagnosis of metastatic disease is 18-24 months, but this varies widely between patients.

Clinical patterns of relapse predict future behaviour. Patients with a long interval without disease (more than two years) after primary diagnosis and favourable sites of recurrence (such as local lymph nodes and chest wall) survive longer than patients with either a short interval without disease or recurrence at other sites. Patients with visceral disease have the poorest outlook; these patients tend to have a short interval without disease and have cancers that are biologically more aggressive.

Treatment of metastatic disease

Hormonal treatment of metastatic breast cancer

Premenopausal women
- Oophorectomy
- Radiation menopause
- Gonadotrophin releasing hormone analogues
- Other treatments as for postmenopausal women

Postmenopausal women
- Tamoxifen (or pure antioestrogen when available)
- Aromatase inhibitors (such as aminoglutethimide and 4-hydroxyandrostenedione)
- New oral aromatase inhibitors (currently in clinical trials)
- Progestogens (such as medroxyprogesterone acetate and megestrol acetate)

Antioestrogens, aromatase inhibitors, and progestogens may be used in virtually any sequence in responsive patients.

A patient may present with metastatic breast carcinoma or develop a systemic recurrence after treatment for an apparently localised breast cancer. The aim of treatment is to produce effective control of symptoms with minimal side effects. In terms of drug treatment this ideal is only achieved by hormonal treatment in the 30% of patients whose cancers respond to such drugs. There is no evidence that treating patients with asymptomatic metastases improves overall survival, and chemotherapy should be given routinely only to symptomatic patients.

Doses and side effects of hormonal treatments for metastatic disease

Aromatase inhibitors

Aminoglutethimide
Dose: 250 mg daily without hydrocortisone
Side effects: skin rash, somnolence
These side effects are less common now that the drug is given in a lower dose and without hydrocortisone.

4-Hydroxyandrostenedione
Dose: 250 mg given intramuscularly every two weeks
Side effects: local reactions

Progestogens

Megestrol acetate
Dose: 160 mg daily

Medroxyprogesterone acetate
Dose: 500 mg to 1 g daily
Side effects: hirsutism, weight gain, break through vaginal bleeding (spotting)

Hormonal treatment

A variety of hormonal drugs is available for use in metastatic breast cancer. Objective responses to hormonal treatment are seen in 30% of all patients and in 50-60% of patients with oestrogen receptor positive tumours. Response rates of 25% are seen with second line hormonal treatments, although less than 15% of patients who show no response to first line hormonal treatment will respond to second line treatment, and 10-15% respond to third line treatment.

Chemotherapy

With chemotherapy, a balance must be made between achieving a high rate of response and limiting the side effects. The best palliation is obtained with regimens that produce the highest response rates. Overall rates of response to chemotherapy are about 40-60%, with a median time to relapse of six to 10 months. Subsequent courses of chemotherapy have lower rates of response of less than 25%. The chemotherapy regimens used for metastatic breast cancer are similar to those used for adjuvant and primary systemic treatment. Analogues of the most potent drug (doxorubicin) are commonly used in metastatic breast cancer, but there is no evidence to favour their use in routine practice.

Metastatic breast cancer

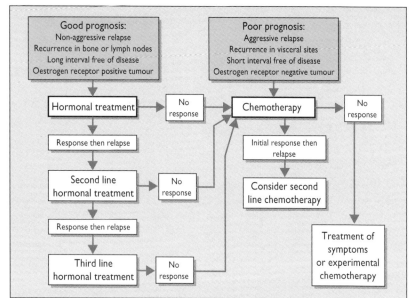

Good prognosis:	Poor prognosis:
Non-aggressive relapse	Aggressive relapse
Recurrence in bone or lymph nodes	Recurrence in visceral sites
Long interval free of disease	Short interval free of disease
Oestrogen receptor positive tumour	Oestrogen receptor negative tumour

Choices of treatment for metastatic or recurrent breast cancer.

High dose chemotherapy—New technologies, including the use of growth factors to stimulate regeneration of bone marrow and the detection and culture of blood progenitor cells, have encouraged research into high dose chemotherapy above the amounts normally tolerated by bone marrow. The main life threatening complication of this approach is bone marrow aplasia. Short term results from high dose chemotherapy for metastatic breast cancer look promising, with 15-20% of selected patients remaining free of disease after three to 10 years. However, long term controlled studies are needed to compare this method with the best standard treatments before its use becomes widespread, and its role is currently limited to experimental work in a few centres.

Specific problems

Treatment of bone metastases

Localised bone pain
- External beam radiotherapy
- Analgesics including opiates
- Non-steroidal anti-inflammatory drugs

Widespread bone pain
- Radioactive strontium
- Sequential hemibody radiotherapy
- Analgesics including opiates
- Non-steroidal anti-inflammatory drugs

Pathological fractures*
- Internal fixation and radiotherapy

*Also prophylactic treatment for patients at risk of fracture.

Bone disease

The bony skeleton is a site of symptomatic disease in three quarters of patients who develop secondary breast cancer. The complications of this are therefore of considerable importance. Widespread bone disease often responds well to hormonal treatment, but in young patients cytotoxic agents may be required. Measuring the benefit of anticancer drug treatment in terms of objective regression of tumour may be difficult, with bone scans being unreliable as indicators of response to treatment. For this reason, measurement of tumour markers may be of use in assessing response in bony metastatic disease.

Localised bone pain should be treated by radiotherapy: a single dose is often all that is required. For patients with more widespread disease or recurrence in previously irradiated areas, alternative measures are required. Analgesic drugs are the mainstay of treatment, either as a prelude to effective anticancer treatment or as a long term alternative or supplement to this treatment. Non-steroidal anti-inflammatory drugs are surprisingly potent in dealing with bone pain, even compared with opiates. Combining the two classes of drugs increases efficacy while minimising side effects.

Widespread bone pain may also be treated by radioactive strontium with few systemic side effects or by sequential upper and lower hemibody radiotherapy. The latter treatment is associated with more toxicity (for example, nausea and vomiting). Bisphosphonates for diffuse bone pain also appear to be effective, although their true role remains to be determined.

Radiographs showing metastatic lesions in humerus (left) and changes after course of hormonal treatment with consequent reduction in bone pain (right).

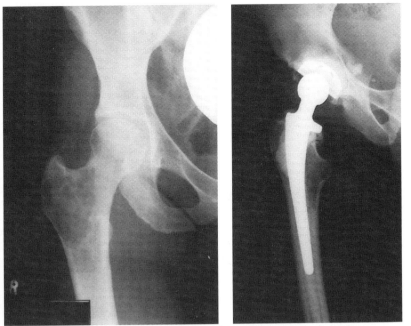

Radiographs showing lytic lesion in neck of femur (left) and prophylactic replacement (right). (Patient was alive, well, and fully mobile three years later.)

Pathological fractures due to bone metastases should be avoided and can be predicted by a sharp increase in pain over a few days or weeks. When bone lysis threatens fracture, internal fixation followed by radiotherapy (low dose in a few fractions) will improve quality of life and mobility and can be associated with a reasonable survival. If a pathological fracture does occur the same combination of internal fixation and radiotherapy should be used, but the functional result is inferior to that of prophylactic treatment.

Marrow infiltration

Any of the peripheral blood elements may be reduced by marrow infiltration, but a "leucoerythroblastic picture" (immature cells in the peripheral blood) suggests extensive marrow infiltration. Chemotherapy is generally required and should be given initially in reduced doses with careful monitoring and adequate supportive care.

Malignant pleural effusion

Up to half of patients with metastatic breast cancer will develop a malignant pleural effusion, but only some of these will require specific treatment. Cytological examination of effusion fluid is positive for malignant cells in over 85% of patients. Aspiration of fluid alone is ineffective in controlling malignant pleural effusions, and 97-100% of patients reaccumulate fluid. In contrast, tube drainage alone is effective in controlling effusions in just over a third of patients. For most patients, however, installation of bleomycin, tetracycline, talc, or inactivated *Corynebacterium parvum* is required to control recurrence. All are relatively safe, with the main problems being pain, which is usually transient, and pyrexia.

Treatment of hypercalcaemia in breast cancer
Hydration
Bisphosphonates
Mobilisation
Anticancer treatment

Malignant hypercalcaemia

The treatment of this complication has been transformed by the availability of bisphosphonates, and these are the agents of choice after hydration with saline (about 3 litres given over 24 hours). Hypercalcaemia is nearly always symptomatic if the blood calcium concentration is more than 3 mmol/l after effective hydration. Effective anticancer treatment reduces the risk of recurrence, but patients whose disease is refractory to this treatment and who exhibit continuing hypercalcaemia can be treated with intravenous bisphosphonates given every two to four weeks. Oral bisphosphonates are available, and their role in recurrent hypercalcaemia is being investigated.

Neurological complications

Although non-metastatic syndromes of the central nervous system can occur with breast cancer, any focal neurological symptom must be investigated. Computed tomography or magnetic resonance imaging can detect even small volumes of disease in the brain. Isotope brain scanning is unhelpful. Cord disease is best detected by magnetic resonance imaging or computed tomography. The initial treatment of brain metastases is to reduce oedema with high dose corticosteroids (12-16 mg daily of dexamethasone) pending local treatment with fractionated radiotherapy. Radiotherapy produces most benefit in patients whose neurological symptoms improve after taking steroids. Radiotherapy may be given in just five fractions. The long term results of treating disease of the central nervous system are disappointing, with most patients dying within three to four months. Long term survival may occur in patients with a solitary metastasis if there is no evidence of involvement of visceral sites and the disease is hormone responsive. Depending on the site, some of these patients are best treated by excision of the metastasis followed by postoperative radiotherapy and appropriate systemic treatment.

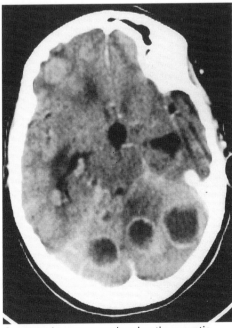

Computed tomogram showing three cystic metastases in cerebellum and one metastasis in frontal lobe.

Metastatic breast cancer

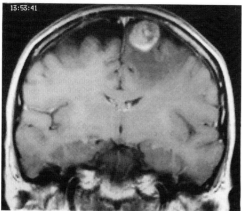

Enhanced magnetic resonance image showing isolated metastasis in fronto-parietal region. In the absence of any other disease, this is suitable for treatment by excision and postoperative radiotherapy.

Cord compression is not usually amenable to surgery and is seen most often in patients with thoracic spinal metastases. Treatment with steroids and fractionated radiotherapy (5-10 treatments) may produce dramatic responses provided that treatment is started as soon as possible and before neurological deficits (paraparesis and bladder and bowel dysfunction) are severe. Patients with isolated metastases causing cord compression who are fit can be treated by emergency laminectomy. Infiltration or compression of nerves (such as infiltration of the brachial plexus) by a tumour may produce pain, paresis, and paraesthesia. Palliative radiotherapy helps but analgesic drugs, often in combination with amitriptyline or mexiletine, may be required.

Control of pain

Choice of analgesic for control of pain

	Class of analgesic	Preferred drug
Mild pain	Simple analgesic	Paracetamol (preferable to aspirin because of lack of gastrointestinal side effects)
Moderate pain	Weak opioid analgesic (alone or in combination with simple analgesic)	Co-proxamol or codeine with paracetamol
Severe pain	Strong opioid analgesic	Morphine

Adjuvant drugs for control of pain

Cause of pain	Useful adjuvant drug
Soft tissue infiltration	Non-steroidal anti-inflammatory drugs
	Prednisolone*
Hepatic enlargement	Prednisolone*
Raised intracranial pressure	Dexamethasone†
Compression or infiltration of nerves	Dexamethasone†
	Amitriptyline
	Carbamazepine
	Mexiletine
Muscle spasm	Diazepam
	Baclofen
Fungating tumour	Antibiotics
	Systemic co-amoxiclav or metronidazole
	Topical metronidazole
Cellulitis	Systemic antibiotics

*Dose of 30-40 mg daily; withdraw if no effect in two weeks.
†Initial dose of 12-16 mg daily, gradually reducing dose to minimum required for control of symptoms.

Control of other symptoms in patients with metastatic breast cancer

Symptom	Treatment
Anorexia	Prednisolone or progestogens
Dysphagia	Antifungal drugs if related to candidiasis
	External beam irradiation, surgical intubation, or endoscopic laser treatment if mechanical evidence of obstruction
	Consider chemotherapy if dysphagia due to mediastinal node compression
Nausea and vomiting	Treat underlying cause
	Antiemetics (such as metoclopramide or cyclizine) with or without prednisolone
Constipation	Laxatives
Dyspnoea	Morphine and benzodiazepines
Cough	Codeine or methadone linctus or morphine oral solution
	Nebulised local anaesthetics

About 60-70% of patients with metastatic breast cancer complain of pain. These patients rarely have one site of pain, and most have several pains that may have different causes. Each site of pain and the mechanism underlying the pain should be identified. Patients' emotional states (anger, despair, fear, anxiety, or depression) may be important in relation to how they respond to their pain and need to be assessed and treated as part of their pain.

Analgesia should be simple and flexible and appropriate for the severity of the pain. If simple or weak opioid analgesics do not bring the pain under control quickly, treatment with strong opioid analgesics or adjuvant drugs should be started. Laxatives should be given to patients treated with opiates to prevent constipation. Some drugs have no intrinsic analgesic activity but can contribute significantly to pain control when used in combination with analgesics. Anxiety, restlessness, and insomnia may be treated with benzodiazepines: diazepam is the preferred oral anxiolytic, temazepam is the hypnotic of choice, and midazolam the drug of choice for parenteral use. The place of antidepressants in the management of chronic pain is not clear, but some patients with advanced or terminal malignant disease do seem to respond to them.

Patients with breast cancer also have other symptoms that require treatment, including anorexia, dysphagia, nausea and vomiting, respiratory symptoms, headache, and malodour.

While it may not be possible to cure or prolong the lives of some patients with metastatic breast cancer, much can be done to improve their quality of life. Management of cancer patients with end stage disease should be multidisciplinary and include palliative care physicians or physicians with an interest in treating pain. Control of symptoms is only one aspect of palliative care, and the resources of a skilled multidisciplinary team are needed to ensure that the psychological and social problems of patients and their family are appropriately addressed.

The computed tomogram was supplied by Dr Andrew Wright and the magnetic resonance image by Dr Rod Gibson; both are radiologists at Western General Hospital, Edinburgh.

PROGNOSTIC FACTORS

W R Miller, I O Ellis, J R C Sainsbury

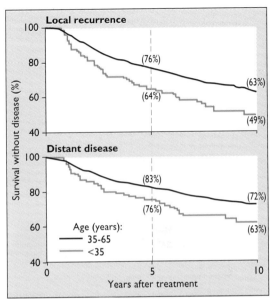

Freedom from recurrence of cancer in patients in relation to age when breast cancer first diagnosed. (Proportional hazards model showed age <35 to have relative risk of 1·6 for distant disease.)

Prognostic factors are of value for three main reasons:
- To help select the appropriate treatment for individual patients
- To allow comparisons of treatments between groups of patients at similar risks of recurrence or death
- To improve our understanding of breast cancer, which may permit the development of new strategies or treatments

Prognostic factors can be broadly classified into two groups: chronological factors, which are indicators of how long the cancer has been present and relate to stage of disease at presentation, and biological factors, which relate to the intrinsic or potential behaviour of the tumour. However, recent evidence suggests that age at diagnosis may also be a risk factor: younger women (aged under 35) have a poorer prognosis than older patients with cancer of equivalent stage.

Chronological factors

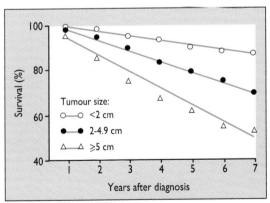

Survival in relation to size of breast cancer.

Tumour size

The pathological size of a tumour correlates directly with survival; patients with smaller tumours have a better survival rate than those with large tumours. Maximum pathological size should be assessed in fresh specimens, and the size should be subsequently confirmed or amended after histological examination.

Status of axillary lymph nodes

The single best prognostic factor is the presence or absence of axillary nodal metastases. There is a direct correlation between survival and the number of axillary lymph nodes involved.

Metastases

Patients in whom cancer has spread beyond the axillary or internal mammary nodes (M_1 or stage IV disease) have a much worse survival rate than patients whose disease is apparently localised. There are differences in survival between patients depending on the site of the metastatic disease, with patients who have supraclavicular involvement as their only site of metastases having a much better survival rate than patients with metastases at other sites.

Survival of patients with breast cancer according to involvement of axillary lymph nodes

	Survival at 10 years
All patients	45·9%
Negative axillary lymph nodes	64·9%
Positive axillary lymph nodes:	24·9%
1-3	37·5%
≥4	13·4%

Survival of patients according to stage of tumour

Stage	Survival at 5 years
I	84%
II	71%
III	48%
IV	18%

Biological factors

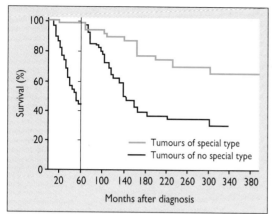

Short and long term survival in relation to histological type of breast cancer.

Survival of patients according to histological grade of tumour

Histological grade	Survival at 10 years
I	85%
II	60%
III	40%

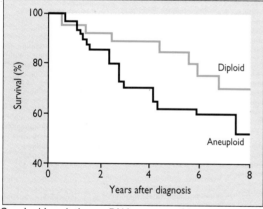

Survival in relation to DNA content of breast cancer.

Biochemical measurements

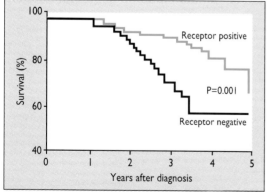

Survival in relation to concentration of oestrogen receptor in breast cancer.

Histological type

Many of the so called special types of invasive breast carcinoma (invasive tubular, cribriform, mucinous, papillary, and microinvasive) are associated with a much better prognosis than cancers of no special type. Histological type is one of the best predictors of long term survival.

Histological grade

The three characteristics of tubular formation, nuclear pleomorphism, and mitotic frequency are assessed in a semiquantitative manner to give three histological grades (I, II, and III) which correlate directly with survival. Grade should be assessed on well fixed specimens, which for most tumours means that the carcinoma should be sliced while fresh to allow rapid penetration of fixative.

Lymphatic or vascular invasion

Tumour cells can be identified in lymphatic and blood vessels in up to a quarter of all patients with breast cancer. Their presence is associated with a doubling of the rate of local recurrence after wide local excision or mastectomy, and patients with this feature are at high risk of short term systemic relapse.

Markers of proliferation

Patients with tumours that have a high rate of proliferation have an increased rate of local recurrence and a worse survival rate than patients whose tumours proliferate slowly. Several methods to measure proliferation have been reported, including measurement of the fraction of cells in the S phase of the cell cycle; the use of monoclonal antibodies such as Ki67, KiS1, and MIB-1; and identification of proliferating cells by the use of tracers such as bromodeoxyuridine. Measurement of proliferation alone does not give complete information about a tumour because in each tumour there is a balance between proliferation and cell loss and because prognosis depends not only on the rate of proliferation but also on the metastatic potential of a breast cancer.

DNA content of a tumour

Normal cells are diploid with regard to their DNA content. Many breast cancers have abnormal amounts of DNA and are aneuploid. Patients with aneuploid breast cancers have a much worse prognosis than those with diploid tumours.

Hormone and growth factor receptors

The presence of oestrogen receptors in a breast cancer predicts response to hormonal manipulation; this appears to be of some value in predicting early outcome after treatment but is of limited value in predicting long term survival. Progesterone receptors can be identified in some breast cancers; their presence depends on an intact oestrogen receptor pathway, but it is not clear that they are of more value than oestrogen receptors in predicting prognosis or response to hormonal treatment.

The presence of epidermal growth factor receptors within the membrane of breast cancer cells is inversely correlated with the presence of oestrogen receptors and is associated with a diminished period free of relapse and reduced overall survival. Patients whose tumours are positive for epidermal growth factor receptors are unlikely to respond to hormonal treatment. The possibility of using this growth factor receptor pathway as a target for treating breast cancers is currently being investigated.

Oncogenes

The proto-oncogene erbB2 is overexpressed in 15-30% of invasive cancers and in up to 80% of non-invasive cancers, and its product is homologous with the epidermal growth factor receptor. Patients with lymph node involvement whose tumours express erbB2 have a particularly poor prognosis, but erbB2 seems to be of less value in delineating the prognosis of patients who are lymph node negative. Tumours which express erbB2 are more likely to be resistant to both chemotherapy and hormonal treatment.

Tumour suppressor genes

p53 Is a product of a gene found on the short arm of chromosome 17. Its abnormal expression is the most common genetic lesion detected in breast cancers, and one group of patients who have a greatly increased risk of breast, ovarian, and bowel cancer (those with Li-Fraumeni syndrome) have abnormal p53 expression. The product of the gene seems to be a transcription factor responsible for checking the fidelity of cell replication.

Proteases

Cathepsin D is a protease capable of degrading basement membrane. It is not clear whether the cathepsin D found in breast cancers is primarily derived from malignant cells or from macrophages. Early studies suggested that the presence of cathepsin D in a tumour correlated with prognosis, but recent studies have failed to confirm this.

Second messenger systems

Cyclic AMP binding proteins are the regulatory subunits of a major second messenger system—protein kinase A. High concentrations of cyclic AMP binding proteins are present in 10-15% of breast cancers, and patients with these cancers have a very poor survival rate. The concentration of cyclic AMP binding protein can be used to identify a subgroup of patients who do not have axillary node involvement but yet have a very poor outlook.

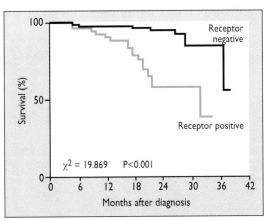

Survival in relation to concentration of epidermal growth factor receptor in breast cancer.

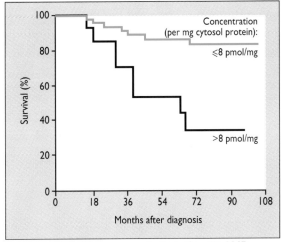

Survival of patients with breast cancer and involved axillary lymph nodes in relation to expression of oncogene erbB2.

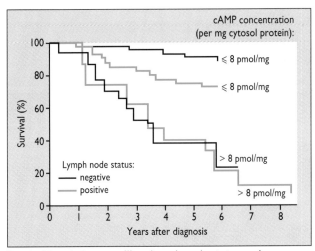

Survival in relation to concentration of cyclic AMP binding proteins in breast cancer.

Survival in relation to axillary lymph node status and concentration of cyclic AMP binding proteins in breast cancer.

Use of prognostic factors

Nottingham prognostic index=
(0·2×size)+lymph node stage+grade

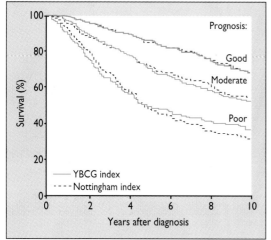

Survival of patients with breast cancer according to Nottingham and Yorkshire Breast Cancer Group prognostic indices.

Interrelated factors

Many of the factors which correlate with outcome are interrelated and do not therefore have independent prognostic significance. For example, grade III tumours are likely to be oestrogen receptor negative, to be epidermal growth factor receptor positive, have a high proliferative index, and to be aneuploid. When a multivariate analysis is performed and histological grade is entered first, little further prognostic information is obtained by entering these other factors. Measurements of large numbers of prognostic factors is therefore of no value in the routine management of patients with breast cancer.

Prognostic indices

Although individual factors are useful, combining independent prognostic variables in the form of an index allows identification of groups of patients with different prognoses. The Nottingham prognostic index is the most widely used index and incorporates three prognostic factors: tumour size, node status, and histological grade.

With the Nottingham index the lymph node stage is 1 if no nodes are involved, 2 if one to three nodes are involved, and 3 if four or more nodes are involved. The Yorkshire Breast Cancer Group categorised lymph node stage as 1 if no nodes were involved or 3 for any axillary node involvement. The Yorkshire group also used different codes for tumour grade: code 1 for grade I and code 2 for grades II and III. Both indices identify three prognostic groups. The good prognostic group has a survival similar to that of age matched controls without breast cancer, and such women are unlikely to benefit from aggressive forms of adjuvant treatment. In contrast the poor prognostic group, with a 13% survival after 15 years, may well benefit from more intensive systemic treatment.

The sources of the data presented in the graphs are: A J Nixon *et al*, *J Clin Oncol* 1994;**12**:888-94 for disease free survival in relation to age; C L Carter *et al*, *Cancer* 1989;**63**:181-7 for survival in relation to cancer size; O-P Kallioniemi *et al*, *Br J Cancer* 1987;**56**:637-42 for survival in relation to DNA content; R A Hawkins *et al*, *Br J Surg* 1987;**74**:1009-13 (Blackwell Science) for survival in relation to oestrogen receptor status; J R C Sainsbury *et al*, *Lancet* 1987;i:1398-402 (copyright the Lancet) for survival in relation to epidermal growth factor receptor status; A K Tandon, *J Clin Oncol* 1989;**7**:1120-8 for survival in relation to erbB2 expression; W R Miller *et al*, *Br J Cancer* 1990;**61**: 263-6 for survival in relation to cyclic AMP binding protein concentration; W R Miller *et al*, *Breast Cancer Res Treat* 1993;**26**:89-94 (Kluwer Academic Publishers) for survival in relation to lymph node status and cyclic AMP binding protein concentration; and J M Brown *et al*, *The Breast* 1993;**2**:144-7 for survival according to prognostic indices. The data are reproduced with permission of the journals or publishers.

CLINICAL TRIALS OF MANAGEMENT OF BREAST CANCER

D Riley, M Baum

Importance of clinical trials

Clinical trials provide a reliable way to evaluate the efficacy of new treatments. When a new treatment is overwhelmingly superior to all previous treatments, as was the case when antibiotics were introduced, clinical trials are not necessary. Most new treatments, however, require rigorous testing to demonstrate their superiority (or not) over current optimal management. To eliminate bias and to ensure that treatment groups are comparable, randomisation is required and is a key component of clinical trials.

With a disease as common as breast cancer a small improvement in survival of the order of 5% would translate into many thousands of lives saved worldwide. Large multicentre trials are necessary to demonstrate such an effect. For example, detection of an improvement in five year survival from 55% to 60% with 90% power at the 5% level would require 4100 patients, and detection of this difference with 95% power would require over 5000 patients. Data from different trials can be combined for meta-analysis to increase confidence that even small effects of treatments on outcome will be detected. Most clinical trials have evaluated different treatments in operable breast cancer and can be considered as four specific categories.

Categories of treatments for breast cancer investigated by clinical trials

- Extent of surgical treatment
- Role of postoperative radiotherapy
- Role of hormonal treatments
- Role of chemotherapy

Extent of surgery

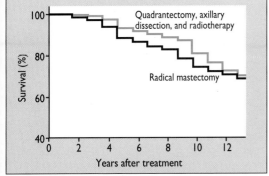

Survival of patients with breast cancer treated by quadrantectomy, axillary dissection, and radiotherapy or by radical mastectomy.

Early trials compared radical mastectomy (total removal of breast and both pectoral muscles) with supraradical procedures (removal of breast; of axillary, supraclavicular, internal mammary, and mediastinal nodes; and of thymus). No survival advantage was evident for the more extensive surgery. Trials to evaluate whether there was an alternative to mastectomy were started in the 1960s and '70s. One study from Milan compared radical mastectomy with removal of the quadrant of the breast in which the tumour was situated (quadrantectomy) combined with postoperative radiotherapy to the breast. Overall survival and survival without relapse were identical with the two treatments.

Subsequent studies have shown that less extensive local resections (wide local excision) followed by whole breast radiotherapy provide similar rates of local control and survival to that seen with quadrantectomy or total mastectomy (removal of the breast without removal of pectoralis major muscle). Any local resection must adequately excise both the invasive and associated non-invasive cancer (clear histological margins) to achieve satisfactory rates of local control. Wide local excision has the advantage that the cosmetic result is superior to that of quadrantectomy. Trials have shown that patients undergoing breast conserving treatments suffer similar psychological morbidity to those patients undergoing mastectomy; patients treated by breast conservation do, however, report greater freedom of dress and better body image than patients treated by mastectomy.

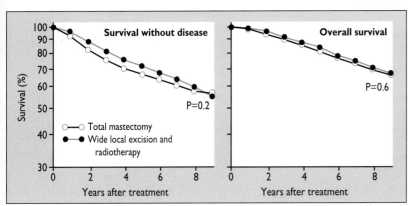

Survival without disease and overall survival of breast cancer patients treated by wide local excision and radiotherapy or by total mastectomy.

Summary results of trials of primary surgery for breast cancer

- Extent of local surgery does not appear to influence survival
- Failure of treatment or local recurrence is often a result of poor prognosis rather than a cause of it
- Breast conservation surgery should be supplemented with radiotherapy
- Locoregional control (control in the axilla and breast) is important
- All patients require similar psychological support regardless of the extent of surgery

---

Some trials have compared the roles of surgery and radiotherapy in the control of axillary nodal disease. Most have shown that a full level III clearance of axillary nodes results in a lower rate of axillary relapse than axillary radiotherapy. Both axillary clearance and axillary radiotherapy, however, convey no benefit to patients who are axillary node negative, which is now the case for the majority of patients presenting for treatment with breast cancer. Although the extent of axillary surgery is important in relation to local relapse and provision of adequate prognostic information, neither axillary surgery nor radiotherapy appear to have any influence on overall survival.

Role of radiotherapy

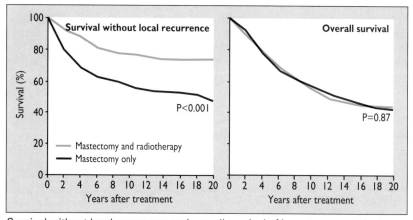

Survival without local recurrence and overall survival of breast cancer patients treated by mastectomy alone or by mastectomy and chest wall radiotherapy.

Early trials compared the combination of mastectomy and postoperative radiotherapy with radical mastectomy. Locoregional recurrences were seen less often in patients treated by radiotherapy. Subsequent trials compared total mastectomy with or without postoperative radiotherapy and have confirmed that radiotherapy reduces the rate of local recurrence but has no apparent effect on overall survival. Analysis of patients in these trials has allowed identification of risk factors for local recurrence, which can now be used to select patients who would benefit from chest wall radiotherapy after mastectomy.

Trials have shown that local control is improved by whole breast radiotherapy after breast conserving treatment. Studies are currently under way to determine whether it is necessary to give radiotherapy to patients with tumours that have been detected by breast screening and that are small, node negative, well differentiated, or of special type. An overview of data from early radiotherapy trials suggested that radiotherapy had a detrimental effect on long term survival, but a more recent analysis that included patients treated with more modern equipment and techniques did not show this.

Role of hormonal treatments

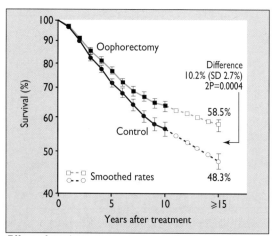

Effect of oophorectomy on survival of breast cancer patients aged under 50.

Ovarian ablation

Early studies gave conflicting results on the value of ovarian ablation, and, with the introduction of chemotherapy, the role of adjuvant ovarian ablation was largely ignored. The benefits of oophorectomy only became evident after a meta-analysis of these trials, which showed that ovarian ablation in premenopausal women (aged <50) produced an improvement in survival of the same order as that achieved by polychemotherapy.[1] Oophorectomy appears to produce greatest benefits in patients with breast cancer that is oestrogen receptor positive.

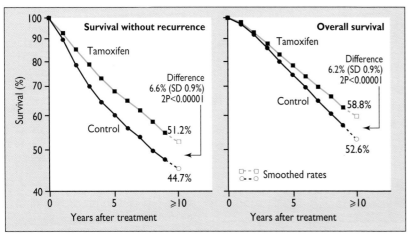

Effect of tamoxifen on survival without recurrence and overall survival of breast cancer patients.

Tamoxifen

Trials have shown a significant improvement in survival free from disease and overall survival for patients receiving tamoxifen.[1] Most trials have restricted entry to postmenopausal patients, but results also show a survival benefit for premenopausal women. Trials are currently under way to determine the appropriate length of treatment with tamoxifen; data indicate that two years of tamoxifen treatment is better than one, but whether five or more years of treatment produce a significantly greater benefit is still being assessed. Tamoxifen is of greatest benefit in patients with oestrogen receptor positive tumours, but it also produces a smaller but still significant survival advantage for patients with oestrogen receptor negative tumours.[1] Since the rate of relapse is greater in patients with receptor negative tumours, however, the absolute benefits for patients with oestrogen receptor positive and receptor negative tumours are similar.

Trials of tamoxifen have also shown a 39% reduction in the incidence of contralateral carcinomas in patients taking this drug.[1] These findings have been the basis of the recent tamoxifen prevention trials. One trial has shown that tamoxifen may reduce deaths from heart disease, which is consistent with the reduction in cholesterol concentrations produced by tamoxifen.

Effect of tamoxifen on mortality in postmenopausal women with breast cancer

Oestrogen receptor concentration of primary breast cancer (fmol/mg cytosol protein)	% Reduction in annual odds of death (SD)
Poor (<10 fmol/mg)	16 (6)
Positive (>10 fmol/mg)	23 (4)
Unknown	17 (4)

Role of chemotherapy

Effect of polychemotherapy on survival of breast cancer patients.

Trials of perioperative chemotherapy, in which a short but intensive course of chemotherapy was given at the time of surgery, showed early promise. Subsequent trials have not confirmed an improvement in survival with this treatment. Studies of postoperative polychemotherapy show a consistent 25% reduction in relative risk of death for up to 10 years.[1] The absolute gain depends on the risk of a particular group of patients: absolute benefit may range from one event saved in 100 patients with a good prognosis to 10 events saved in 100 patients with a poor prognosis.

Projected benefit of adjuvant treatment for patients with breast cancer according to prognosis

	Prognosis of patients	
	Poor	Very good
Probability of 10 year survival without adjuvant treatment	60%	96%
Probability of dying	40%	4%
Reduction in odds of death by adjuvant treatment	25%	25%
Absolute benefit from treatment	10%	1%
Projected 10 year survival after treatment	70%	97%

Effect of age and menopausal status on mortality after polychemotherapy

Age (years)	Menopausal status	% Reduction in annual odds of death (SD)
<50	Premenopausal	25 (6)
50-59	Premenopausal	23 (9)
50-59	Postmenopausal	13 (7)
60-69	Either	10 (6)

When a treatment is non-toxic and easy to administer, then even a 1% absolute benefit is worth while, but chemotherapy is toxic so that the benefits must be balanced against the risks. Several trials are currently addressing the question of who should receive chemotherapy. Chemotherapy appears to have the greatest effect on survival in younger, premenopausal women.[1]

Clinical trials of management of breast cancer

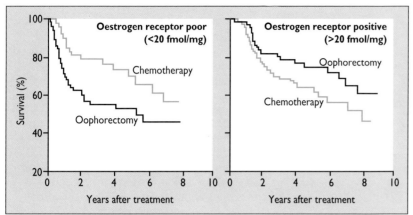

Survival without recurrence of breast cancer patients treated by oophorectomy or chemotherapy in relation to oestrogen receptor content of tumour.

Few trials have tried to determine which premenopausal women should be treated by oophorectomy and which should be treated by chemotherapy. A recent trial has suggested that patients who have tumours that are oestrogen receptor positive show greater benefit after ovarian manipulation whereas patients with oestrogen receptor negative tumours do better after chemotherapy. Data from meta-analysis indicate that improvements in survival obtained by hormone manipulation and chemotherapy may be additive, particularly in postmenopausal women.[1] The effects of adding the two treatments in premenopausal women is not at all clear, and several trials are investigating this.

No data are yet available from randomised trials comparing surgery followed by adjuvant treatment with initial systemic treatment followed by local treatments (surgery or radiotherapy).

Trials in elderly patients

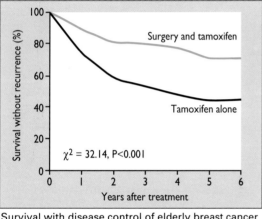

Survival with disease control of elderly breast cancer patients treated by tamoxifen alone or by surgery and tamoxifen.

Uncontrolled series of patients treated by tamoxifen alone in the 1970s suggested that patients aged over 70 could be adequately treated this way. Subsequent randomised trials have shown that better rates of local control can be obtained with a combination of surgery and tamoxifen rather than tamoxifen alone. Ongoing trials are investigating whether selecting patients on the basis of tumours that are oestrogen receptor positive and responsive to tamoxifen can identify a group of elderly patients who could achieve long term control of disease by taking tamoxifen alone.

Further trials

Topics of current and future trials

- Is primary systemic treatment associated with improvements in survival?

- Do combinations of hormonal treatment and chemotherapy produce greater benefits than either treatment alone?

- What is the role of high dose chemotherapy with rescue by bone marrow or stem cells in women at high risk of metastatic recurrence and death?

- Do the new aromatase inhibitors have any role in adjuvant treatment?

- Can patients receive hormone replacement therapy after treatment for breast cancer, and does this increase their risk of recurrence?

- Can molecular and biological markers be used to select appropriate treatment for subsets of patients?

There are several unanswered questions in the treatment of breast cancer, some of which are the subject of ongoing clinical trials. Some units have introduced primary systemic treatment for patients with breast cancer, and trials are under way to determine whether primary systemic treatment is associated with better survival rates than surgery followed by appropriate adjuvant systemic treatment. It is important to know whether patients who are at very high risk of death from breast cancer benefit from aggressive regimens of chemotherapy with rescue by bone marrow or stem cells. Trials currently under way in the United Kingdom and United States are addressing this issue.

The sources of the data presented in illustrations are: U Veronesi *et al*, *Eur J Cancer* 1990;**26**: 668-70 for the graph of survival after quadrantectomy or radical mastectomy; B Fisher and C Redmond, *Monogr Natl Cancer Inst* 1992;**11**:7-13 for the graph of survival after wide local excision or total mastectomy; J Houghton *et al*, *World J Surg* 1994;**18**:117-22 (copyright Springer-Verlag) for the graph of survival after mastectomy and radiotherapy or mastectomy only; Early Breast Cancer Triallists' Collaborative Group, *Lancet* 1992;**339**:1-15, 71-85 for the graphs of effects of oophorectomy on survival, effects of tamoxifen on survival, and effects of polychemotherapy on survival and for the table of effect of tamoxifen on mortality; Scottish Cancer Trials Breast Group and ICRF Unit, Guy's Hospital, London, *Lancet* 1993;**341**:1293-8 for the graph of survival after oophorectomy or chemotherapy; and T Bates *et al*, *Br J Surg* 1991;**78**:591-4 (Blackwell Science) for the graph of survival after tamoxifen or tamoxifen and surgery. The data are reproduced with permission of the journals or copyright holders.

1 Early Breast Cancer Triallists' Collaborative Group. Systemic treatment of early breast cancer by hormonal, cytotoxic, or immune therapy. *Lancet* 1992;**339**:1-15,71-85.

PSYCHOLOGICAL ASPECTS

P Maguire

Psychological morbidity

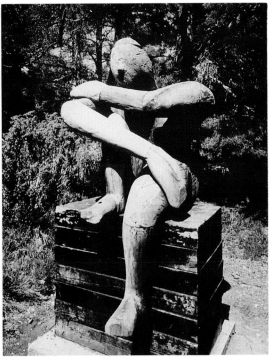

Sculpture of a woman who has had a mastectomy and who is curled up and withdrawn (by Elspeth Bennie).

Most women who present with breast lumps are emotionally distressed. A substantial proportion of women whose lumps prove to be benign remain distressed and may become clinically anxious or depressed, particularly if they suffer from chronic breast pain.

Up to 30% of women with breast cancer develop an anxiety state or depressive illness within a year of diagnosis, which is three to four times the expected rate in matched community samples. After mastectomy 20-30% of patients develop persisting problems with body image and sexual difficulties. Breast conserving surgery reduces problems with body image, but this is offset by increased fears of recurrence. Consequently, the type of surgery does not affect psychiatric morbidity. Immediate breast reconstruction after mastectomy may reduce this morbidity provided that the possible complications have been discussed fully and understood, that the patient wants it for herself and not because of pressure from others, and that it is carried out expertly. Psychiatric morbidity further increases when radiotherapy or chemotherapy is used.

Problems of recognition

Reasons for non-disclosure of psychological morbidity

- Problems are inevitable
- Problems cannot be alleviated
- To avoid burdening health professionals
- To avoid being judged inadequate
- Relevant questions not asked by health professionals
- Cues met by distancing, such as "you are bound to be upset"

Few patients mention psychological morbidity because they do not think that it is acceptable to do so. Doctors can promote disclosure of such problems by asking questions and clarifying the responses about patients' perceptions of the nature of their illness and their reactions to it and about their experience of losing a breast or having radiotherapy or chemotherapy. By being empathic, making educated guesses about how a patient is feeling, and summarising what has been disclosed, doctors promote both disclosure and expression of related feelings.

Disclosure by patients

Inhibited by	*Promoted by*
• Closed questions	• Open directive question
• Leading questions	• Questions with a psychological focus
• Multiple questions	• Clarification of psychological aspects
• Questions with a physical focus	• Summarising
• Offering advice or reassurance especially if premature	• Screening questions
	• Empathy
	• Educated guesses

Disclosure is inhibited by closed, leading, and multiple questions and by giving advice and reassurance, especially if important problems have not been disclosed. If the questions asked in the first few minutes of a consultation focus solely on physical aspects, patients will assume that it is not permissible to discuss other problems. If problems are not disclosed despite encouragement it is useful to ask about the impact of the illness on several key areas: daily functioning since surgery, relationship with a partner, and mood.

Psychological aspects

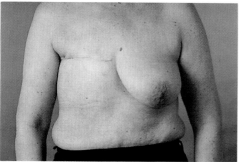

Mastectomy can lead to problems with body image.

When there is any hint of anxiety or depression clinicians should inquire about key symptoms by asking open directive questions—"What changes have you noticed while you have been depressed? How have you been sleeping?" Patients with problems with their body image should be asked how much they avoid looking at their chest wall and how they react if they catch sight of it. With sexual difficulties, clinicians should check whether they represent a new problem and explore the reactions of patients and their partners.

Treatment

Anxiety and depression

Patients who have a core mood change but too few symptoms to justify a clinical diagnosis usually respond to understanding and emotional support and do not merit psychiatric referral, especially given the stigma associated with such a referral.

The treatment of an anxiety state depends on its severity. A patient who is struggling to cope should be given a benzodiazepine (for example, diazepam) to be used as needed for up to three weeks—this avoids the risk of dependency—or a small dose of an antipsychotic drug (for example, thioridazine 25 mg three times a day). Once a patient reports some improvement it is worth teaching them techniques for managing anxiety. This is helpful as further anxiety is often triggered by mention of breast cancer in the media, new physical symptoms, or attendance at clinic. When somatic symptoms of anxiety predominate, the use of a β blocker (for example, propranolol) should be considered.

Depressive illness responds well to antidepressant drugs given in therapeutic doses for four to six months. Doctors should explain that the drugs, unlike tranquillisers, do not cause physical dependence; they reverse the biochemical changes caused by the shock of diagnosis and treatment. Stressing that any other problems will be dealt with once the mood has begun to improve also improves compliance. Agitated patients benefit from a sedating drug (for example, dothiepin, initially 75 mg at night increasing to up to 150 mg). Patients who are apathetic and lethargic benefit from an alerting agent (for example, fluoxetine 20 mg in the morning). If anxiety, depression, or any underlying problems persist psychiatric referral should be considered.

Conditioned responses

Up to a quarter of patients who receive combination chemotherapy develop conditioned responses. Any stimulus that reminds them of treatment causes them to reflexively experience adverse effects like nausea and vomiting. Phobic reactions can develop, which make further chemotherapy difficult. While new antiemetics such as ondansetron have reduced this problem, conditioned responses need to be recognised and treated promptly. Covering each infusion with an anxiolytic drug (for example, lorazepam 2 mg three times a day as needed) for 48 hours before and during treatment is often effective.

Body image and sexual problems

When surgical reconstruction is possible patients must have a chance to talk at length about possible complications as well as advantages and to look at photographs of a range of outcomes. Patients who are ineligible for or who refuse surgery may benefit from graded exposure to views of the chest wall of patients after various procedures or cognitive therapy carried out by a clinical psychologist. Sexual difficulties usually require the attention of a sex therapist.

Criteria for an anxiety state

- Persistent anxiety, tension, or inability to relax
- Present for more than half of the time for four weeks
- Cannot pull self out of it or be distracted by others
- Substantial departure from normal mood

Plus at least four of the following:
- Initial insomnia
- Irritability
- Impaired concentration
- Intolerance of noise
- Panic attacks
- Somatic manifestation

Criteria for depressive illness

- Persistent low mood
- Present for more than half of the time for four weeks
- Cannot be distracted out of it by self or others
- Qualitatively or quantitatively significantly different from normal mood
- Inability to enjoy oneself

Plus at least four of the following:
- Diurnal variation of mood
- Repeated or early waking
- Impaired concentration or indecisiveness
- Feeling hopeless or suicidal
- Feelings of guilt, self blame, being a burden, or worthlessness
- Irritability and anger for no reason
- Loss of interest
- Retardation or agitation

Prevention

Preventing psychological morbidity

- Elicit patient's awareness of diagnosis
- If patient is unaware "test waters" by using euphemisms and tailor statements according to patient's responses
- If patient is aware confirm diagnosis:
  - Pause to let news sink in
  - Acknowledge subsequent distress
  - Establish contributive concerns
  - Check patient's needs for information
  - Give information and advice
  - When appropriate discuss treatment options

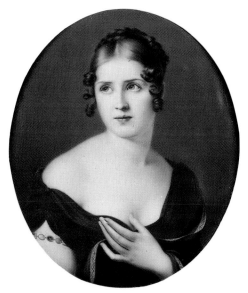

"The Beautiful Greek"—Marie Pauline Bonaparte—by Counis. Marie Pauline, Napoleon's sister, died in 1825 from breast cancer at the age of 45.

Challenging relatives' wishes to withhold diagnosis from patient

- Explore relatives' reasons but respect them
- Establish potential costs to:
  - Relative
  - Key relationship
- Ask permission to check patient's awareness
- If patient is aware confirm diagnosis

Support services

Support measures

- Specialist nurses
- Volunteers
- Self help groups
- National organisations

Breaking bad news

The first step is to check a patient's idea about what is wrong. This will often be that the lump is cancerous. The doctor should confirm that this is correct, pause to let this sink in, acknowledge the patient's distress, and establish what concerns are contributing to this distress. Only then should reassurance, information, and advice be offered. Before doing so, the doctor can ask if the patient has brought someone with her and if she would like this person to be present while her concerns are discussed. Providing tape recordings of the consultation may also facilitate psychological adaptation.

When a patient is unaware that she has cancer the doctor should give a "warning shot" to check if the patient wants to pull out of or move through the process of truth telling. The doctor might say, "The lump is more serious than we thought," and then pause to allow a response such as, "I'll leave the details to you, you're the expert," or, "What do you mean, serious?" The latter type of response indicates a wish to know more, and the doctor should then offer a further euphemism: "The biopsy found some abnormal cells." The patient can pull out of the dialogue or ask for further details. The doctor can then say, "I'm afraid it's cancer," and, after pausing, proceed as described above. This way of breaking bad news reduces the risk of provoking denial or overwhelming distress.

Denial

Some patients will not respond to the warnings about the seriousness of their condition. They wish to remain in denial because the reality is too painful to face. Even so, they will usually ask about treatment. If not, they should be asked whether they would like to know what can be done. When patients reject the need for treatment their denial should be challenged as described in the management of recurrence.

Relatives' views

Relatives may insist that a patient should not be told. They may want to protect her from anguish or believe that she would not cope with the bad news. Their reasons should be explored but respected. They should be invited to reflect on the potential costs to them personally and their relationship and then asked if they would allow the patient's perception of her condition to be explored. If the patient thinks she has breast cancer the doctor should confirm that she is correct and proceed as after breaking bad news. If she is not aware she should be left in denial.

Preference for treatment

It is important to check if a patient has a strong preference for a particular treatment and to honour this when it is technically possible or to explain why it is not feasible. Thus, patients who want to participate in choosing treatment will perceive that the information given is adequate to their needs. Others who want the doctor to decide will not have responsibility thrust upon them. Perceiving the information given to be adequate (neither too much nor too little) protects against anxiety and depression in the short and long term.

Specialist nurses

Specialist nurses can check patients' understanding of and reaction to a consultation when bad news is given and can offer further information and practical and emotional support. There is no firm evidence that such counselling prevents psychological morbidity, but appropriately trained nurses can monitor patients' adjustment and recognise most of those who need help and refer them to a psychologist or psychiatrist. This leads to a fourfold reduction in psychological morbidity. Monitoring each patient once within two months of discharge is as effective as regular monitoring. Patients who develop problems later can be relied on to contact the specialist nurse.

Psychological aspects

Markers of risk for affective disorders

- Past psychiatric illness
- Toxicity due to radiotherapy or chemotherapy
- Lymphoedema or pain
- Problems with body image
- No confiding tie
- Low self esteem
- Unresolved concerns

Names and addresses of self help groups

Breast Cancer Care
- 15-19 Britten Street, London SW3 3TZ
Helpline No (0171) 867 1103
- Suite 2/8, 65 Bath Street, Glasgow G2 2BX
Helpline No (0141) 353 1050
- 9 Castle Terrace, Edinburgh EH1 2DF
Helpline No (0131) 221 0407
- Nationwide Freephone No 0500 245 345

Cancerlink
- 70 Britannia Street, London WC1X 9JN
Telephone No (0171) 833 2451
- 9 Castle Terrace, Edinburgh EH1 2DF
Telephone No (0131) 228 5557
- Asian language line No (0171) 713 7867

British Association of Cancer United Patients
- 3 Bath Place, Rivington Street, London EC2A 3JR
Freephone No 0800 181 199

Leaflets with all national contacts for people with cancer are available from:
Cancer Relief McMillan Fund, Anchor House, 15-19 Britten Street, London SW3 3TZ

Effective training of specialist nurses must ensure that they acquire the skills that promote disclosure and relinquish behaviours that inhibit it. Specialist nurses also need to have regular supervision if they are to remain effective, and they must have rapid access to expert advice from a psychiatrist or clinical psychologist when they uncover severe psychological problems. The use of specialist nurses has disadvantages; other health professionals may leave psychological care to them. Yet it is what treating clinicians say about diagnosis and treatment that is critical in determining patients' psychological adaptation.

Focusing on those at risk—Specialist nurses are most effective if they can identify and concentrate on patients who are at risk of affective disorders. Useful markers of risk have been established, and self rating scales like the hospital anxiety and depression scale or the Rotterdam symptom checklist can also be used to identify probable cases in a clinic.

Volunteers

Patients should be asked if they would like to talk with a volunteer who has been through similar experiences. Appropriately trained volunteers can be contacted through the Breast Cancer Care Group. Alternatively, patients may wish to attend a local self help group. Support groups are helpful providing they are run by people with appropriate experience and sensitivity who are willing to use health professionals as a resource.

Support for the family

It is important to check how a patient's partner and other family members are coping. Many relatives believe that they must not compete with the patient's need for help even though they have as many concerns.

Managing recurrence

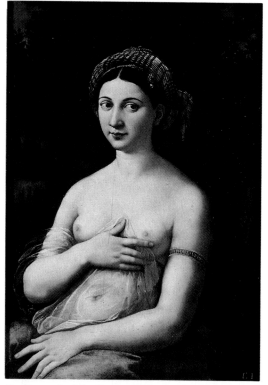

"La Fornarina" by Raphael. The model, Margherita Luti, died young, probably from breast cancer—some think that they can see the stigma of a left breast cancer, which the artist tried to hide.

Some patients are able to put worry about the future to the back of their minds. Others are plagued by uncertainty; their fears should be acknowledged, and they should be asked if they want to know more about their disease status and about signs and symptoms that might herald further deterioration. Negotiating follow up intervals also helps. As long as they remain free of key signs and symptoms such patients cope well, providing they have rapid access to their treating clinician if any develop.

Doctors should avoid agreeing with a relative to withhold a diagnosis of recurrence from a patient. It increases psychiatric disorder and hinders the resolution of the relative's grief. Denial of the gravity of the situation by a patient should be challenged by gently confronting her with inconsistencies—"You say you are better but you are still losing weight"—or by checking if there is a "window" in her denial—"Is there ever a time when you think that it may not work out as well as you hope?"

P Maguire acknowledges the support of the Cancer Research Campaign. The photograph of the sculpture by Elspeth Bennie is reproduced with permission of David Hayes, director of Landmark Highland Heritage and Adventure Park, Carrbridge, Inverness-shire, where the sculpture is sited. The paintings by Counis and Raphael are reproduced by permission of the Bridgeman Art Library.

CARCINOMA IN SITU AND PATIENTS AT HIGH RISK OF BREAST CANCER

D L Page, C M Steel, J M Dixon

Carcinoma in situ

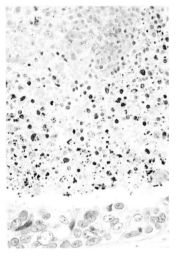

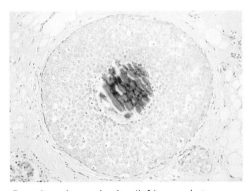

Ductal carcinoma in situ: (left) comedo type carcinoma with extensive necrosis adjacent to viable malignant cells enclosed by basement membrane; (above) with central visible microcalcification.

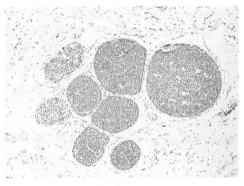

Lobular carcinoma in situ.

Two main types of non-invasive (in situ) cancer can be recognised from the histological pattern of disease and cell type. Ductal carcinoma in situ is the most common form of non-invasive carcinoma (making up 3-4% of symptomatic and 17% of screen detected cancers) and is characterised by ducts and ductules expanded by large irregular cells with large irregular nuclei. In contrast, lobular carcinoma in situ is rare (0·5% of symptomatic and 1% of screen detected cancers) and presents as an expansion of the whole lobule by smaller regular cells with regular, round or oval nuclei.

There has been a lack of agreement among pathologists about whether small lesions should be considered as hyperplasia or in situ carcinoma. In general, lesions that involve only a few membrane bound spaces and that measure less than 2-3 mm in their greatest diameter should be regarded as hyperplastic lesions (with or without atypia) and not in situ carcinoma. There is better agreement about larger lesions.

Classification of ductal carcinoma in situ

Histology	Cytology	Necrosis	Calcification
Comedo	High grade	Extensive	Branched
Intermediate	Intermediate	Limited	Limited
Non-comedo*	Low grade	Absent	Microfoci, inconsistent

*Cribriform, solid, or micropapillary.

Ductal carcinoma in situ

Different classifications of ductal carcinoma in situ have been described, and these correlate to some degree with mammographic patterns of microcalcification.

Presentation—Patients with symptomatic ductal carcinoma in situ present with a breast mass, nipple discharge, or Paget's disease. Screen detected carcinoma is most commonly associated with microcalcification, which may be localised or widespread and is characteristically branching and of variable size and density.

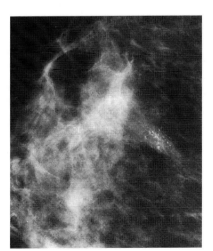

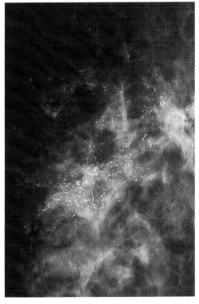

Mammograms showing microcalcification characteristic of ductal carcinoma in situ: localised (left) and widespread (right).

Carcinoma in situ and patients at high risk of breast cancer

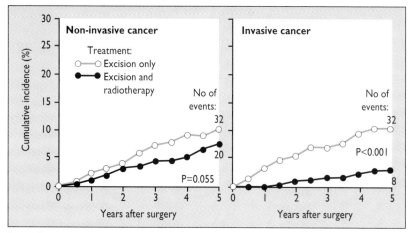

Rate of development of non-invasive and invasive carcinoma after treatment of ductal carcinoma in situ by wide excision alone or wide excision and radiotherapy. (All sizes and types of lesions of ductal carcinoma in situ were included in this study.)

Natural course—Several studies have assessed the risk of subsequent invasive carcinoma in patients in whom ductal carcinoma in situ was missed by the pathologist or the diagnosis was made but mastectomy was not performed. About one third of these patients developed invasive breast cancer in the same breast during follow up of 10-18 years.

Treatment—Symptomatic ductal carcinoma in situ involves much larger areas of the breast than carcinoma in situ detected by screening and has traditionally been treated by mastectomy. Such treatment is associated with excellent long term outcome (98% survival at five years). With the advent of breast screening and the use of conservative surgery for invasive carcinoma, limited surgery has been increasingly used for localised carcinoma in situ. The relative merits of wide excision and mastectomy should be discussed with each patient. Wide excision alone seems to produce satisfactory local control in non-comedo ductal carcinoma in situ (up to 5% recurrence at eight years) but not in comedo carcinoma (30-50% recurrence at eight years). Preliminary data (with follow up of less than four years) from an American study indicate that radiotherapy may reduce the rate of recurrence after excision of a localised area of ductal carcinoma in situ, but it is not clear whether the benefits of radiotherapy relate to all types of ductal carcinoma in situ or whether radiotherapy has any long term adverse effects. Tamoxifen might be expected to reduce the rate of recurrence and the rate of contralateral disease and so may be worth while. Mastectomy is still appropriate treatment for widespread carcinoma in situ; micropapillary ductal carcinoma in situ has a particular tendency to be widespread. Axillary surgery is not indicated in localised ductal carcinoma in situ; but axillary nodal metastases are seen in up to 5% of more widespread disease because of unsuspected microinvasion. Clinical trials are now under way to determine optimum treatment for screen detected ductal carcinoma in situ.

Recommended treatment for ductal carcinoma in situ*

Localised carcinoma in situ (<4 cm)†
- Wide local excision
  Ensure that mammographic lesion has been completely excised with clear histological margins
  Re-excise if margins are involved
  Consider mastectomy if carcinoma >4 cm in size or if micropapillary
- Consider postoperative radiotherapy if comedo type carcinoma
- Consider tamoxifen, 20 mg a day

Widespread carcinoma in situ (≥4 cm)†
- Mastectomy (with or without breast reconstruction)
- Consider tamoxifen

*Outside trials of experimental treatments.
†Extent of carcinoma can be estimated in 80% of patients by measuring extent of malignant microcalcification on mammograms.

Areas of investigation currently being studied in clinical trials

- Natural course of screen detected ductal carcinoma in situ treated by wide excision
- Role of tamoxifen in reducing recurrence after complete excision of localised ductal carcinoma in situ
- Role of radiotherapy in reducing recurrence after complete excision of localised ductal carcinoma in situ

---

Lobular carcinoma in situ

Lobular carcinoma in situ is better defined than ductal carcinoma. Some doctors still use the term lobular neoplasia, which refers to both atypical lobular hyperplasia and lobular carcinoma in situ, largely because of the histological homogeneity of these two conditions. As these lesions have a different natural course, they should be classified separately.

Presentation is often an incidental finding during a breast biopsy and there are no characteristic clinical or mammographic features.

Natural course—About 15-20% of women with a diagnosis of lobular carcinoma in situ will develop breast cancer in the same breast, and a further 10-15% will develop an invasive carcinoma in the contralateral breast.

Treatment—There are three possible approaches: observation, with yearly bilateral mammography; entering the patient into a trial of treatments to prevent breast cancer; or bilateral mastectomy. Bilateral mastectomy should be confined to women who experience severe anxiety that significantly reduces their quality of life. The standard treatment is observation.

Features of ductal and lobular carcinoma in situ

	Ductal carcinoma	Lobular carcinoma
Average age	late 50s	late 40s
Menopausal status	70% postmenopausal	70% premenopausal
Clinical signs	Breast mass, Paget's disease, nipple discharge	None
Mammographic signs	Microcalcification	None
Risk of subsequent carcinoma	30-50% at 10-18 years	25-30% at 15-20 years
Site of subsequent invasive carcinoma:		
Same breast	99%	50-60%
Other breast	1%	40-50%

Patients at high risk of breast cancer

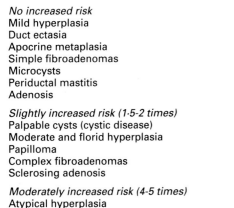

Relative risk of invasive breast cancer associated with benign diseases

No increased risk
Mild hyperplasia
Duct ectasia
Apocrine metaplasia
Simple fibroadenomas
Microcysts
Periductal mastitis
Adenosis

Slightly increased risk (1·5-2 times)
Palpable cysts (cystic disease)
Moderate and florid hyperplasia
Papilloma
Complex fibroadenomas
Sclerosing adenosis

Moderately increased risk (4-5 times)
Atypical hyperplasia

A variety of risk factors have been identified for breast cancer. Factors that are associated with a slightly elevated risk (<2 times) are not clinically relevant and require no specific action. This includes most of the aspects of lifestyle that are risk factors (age at first pregnancy, history of breast feeding, and diet). The only factors associated with significantly increased risks of subsequent breast cancer are certain types of previous benign breast disease and family history.

Previous breast disease

Women with palpable breast cysts, particularly those who develop multiple cysts, and women with certain histological features on biopsy (complex fibroadenomas, duct papillomas, sclerosing adenosis, and moderate or florid usual type hyperplasia) are at some increased risk of breast cancer. However, only women with atypical hyperplasia are at a significantly increased risk. There is an interaction between atypical hyperplasia and family history: women with both atypical hyperplasia and a first degree relative (mother, daughter, or sister) with breast cancer have an absolute risk of 20-30% of developing breast cancer within the next 15-20 years.

Family history

Up to 10% of patients with breast cancer have a genetic abnormality that predisposes them to develop the disease. The presence of a predisposing breast cancer mutation can be suspected from the following:

- Several cases (strictly speaking, a high proportion) of breast cancer in a single family
- Early onset of breast cancer in affected relatives; not all genetically determined breast cancers present in young women, but the earlier the onset the greater the risk that it is genetic
- The presence of multiple epithelial cancers in family members, including bilateral breast cancer or ovarian, colon, and prostate cancer; the combination of breast and ovarian cancers is particularly common in families with a "cancer gene."

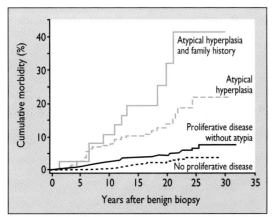

Risk of subsequent development of invasive carcinoma in patients with no epithelial proliferation, proliferative disease without atypia (moderate or florid hyperplasia), atypical hyperplasia, or atypical hyperplasia and a family history of cancer.

Creating a family pedigree—For people who present with a family history of cancer it is necessary to create a family pedigree to confirm that a predisposing mutation is probably present—genetic susceptibility is transmitted as an autosomal dominant trait with limited penetrance—and to estimate the probability that any member of the family has the mutation. The second task is becoming easier as "breast cancer genes" are identified. At present, however, risk is calculated mainly by statistical methods. Word of mouth histories are often inaccurate or incomplete. To assess risk it is necessary to extend and verify details of family histories by examining hospital records; pathology reports; data from cancer registers; and public records of births, marriages, and deaths. Distinctive patterns may then be recognised to allow identification of families carrying a mutation in a particular breast cancer gene such as BRCA1, BRCA2, or p53. In such a family any woman who has not yet developed breast cancer has a less than 50% of chance of carrying the gene, and the risk of having inherited the gene and developing breast cancer decreases as the woman's age increases. For example, if all affected family members developed breast cancer by the age of 45 a female relative aged 55 is unlikely to have inherited the relevant mutation, and her risk of getting breast cancer is little greater than that of the general population.

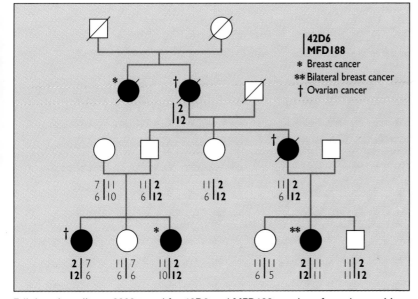

Edinburgh pedigree 2000 typed for 42D6 and MFD188, markers for polymorphism in chromosome 17. All subjects who developed breast or ovarian cancer had the 2/12 pattern of inheritance for the two markers.

Risk of developing breast cancer associated with risk factors

Factors present	Approximate risk
Atypical hyperplasia (specifically defined)	10-15% in next 15-20 years
Atypical hyperplasia and family history of breast cancer*	20-30% in next 15-20 years
Carrier of mutant BRCA1 gene	80-85% during lifetime

*Disease in first degree relative (mother, sister, or daughter).

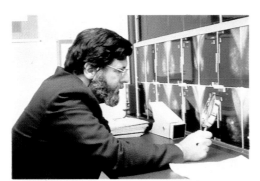

Currently, regular breast screening is limited to women aged 50 or over.

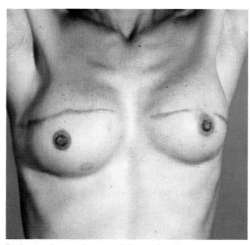

Patient who underwent bilateral subcutaneous mastectomies and immediate breast reconstruction because she was considered to be at very high risk of developing breast cancer.

The source of the data for the graph of rate of development of cancer after excision or excision and radiotherapy is B Fisher *et al*, *N Engl J Med* 1993;**328**:1581-6. The data are reproduced with permission of the journal.

Genetic linkage analysis can be performed if tissue or blood are available from a substantial number of affected members of a family. Such an analysis looks at the inheritance of markers that flank a particular gene, such as the BRCA1 gene on the long arm of chromosome 17. Family members at risk can then be tested for these markers, and marker patterns can be used to assess whether a person is likely to be carrying the affected gene. Genetic linkage is of value principally for women from families carrying a BRCA1 gene mutation. Although this locus is probably involved in only 2% of all breast cancers, it may account for up to 40% of all familial breast cancers. Figures for BRCA2 may be similar. Now that the BRCA1 gene has been cloned, when a precise mutation can be characterised in one affected member of a family, peripheral blood analysis of relatives at risk will identify other carriers of the mutation. Carriers of a mutated breast cancer gene have an 80-85% chance of developing the disease. Genetic analysis is likely to become feasible for BRCA2 and other breast cancer genes in the next few years.

Management of women at high risk

Women at high risk of breast cancer may also be at risk of other cancers, and a coordinated approach to their management is required. Studies have shown that about a third of women with a family history of breast cancer underestimate their own risk by more than half, while a quarter exaggerate their risks by more than this. Many centres now have clinics for women who have a family history of or who are at high risk of breast cancer; these clinics provide the genetic counselling and psychological support that these women need.

There are three possible interventions that might reduce mortality in women at risk:

- Instituting regular screening
- Preventing development of breast cancer
- Performing bilateral subcutaneous mastectomies

Regular screening—As yet there is no evidence that regular screening of high risk groups of women aged under 50 reduces mortality, although randomised studies are presently under way to determine whether screening such women is of value. Current recommendations are that women with a strong family history of breast cancer should be screened by mammography, with screening starting at an age five to 10 years younger than that of the youngest relative to have developed the disease. Ultrasonography is being assessed as a screening tool in younger women, but there is as yet no evidence that it is of value. Nuclear magnetic resonance imaging with computer analysis is also being investigated as a technique that can be repeated regularly to screen high risk women.

Prevention of breast cancer—Studies are under way to assess the value of tamoxifen and retinoids in women at high risk of breast cancer, but the results from these studies will not be available for 10-20 years. Hormonal manipulation by oophorectomy combined with tamoxifen or low dose oestrogen replacement would be expected to reduce the risk of breast cancer while at the same time removing a common site of cancer development (the ovaries) in families in which ovarian cancer and breast cancer are clearly linked. Recent reports indicate that postmenopausal women taking tamoxifen as adjuvant treatment for breast cancer have an increased risk of developing endometrial cancer. Tamoxifen should be used as a preventative treatment only in clinical trials, and patients in such trials should be informed of both the potential risks and benefits.

Bilateral subcutaneous mastectomy performed at five years younger than the youngest family relative to have developed breast cancer might be considered appropriate for women from families that carry the BRCA1 or BRCA2 gene mutations proved by DNA analysis. These operations should be performed by experienced surgeons to ensure that all breast tissue is removed and so that immediate breast reconstruction can be performed.

BREAST RECONSTRUCTION

J D Watson, J R C Sainsbury, J M Dixon

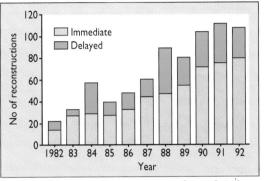

Number of breast reconstructions performed each year for past decade in Edinburgh Breast Unit.

The purpose of the operation is to reconstruct a breast mound to produce breast symmetry. In centres that provide reconstruction there has been a consistent increase in demand, and up to half of patients offered immediate breast reconstruction take up this offer. There is no evidence that immediate reconstruction increases the rate of local or systemic relapse, and it reduces the psychological trauma of the change in body image experienced after mastectomy. Breast reconstruction (particularly immediate reconstruction, which gives substantially better cosmetic and psychological outcomes) should be more widely available than it is at present.

Treatment options

Options for breast reconstruction

Technique	Indications for:	
	Immediate reconstruction	Delayed reconstruction
Prosthesis	Small breasts Adequate skin flaps	As for immediate reconstruction *plus* Well healed scar *plus* No radiotherapy
Tissue expansion and prosthesis	Adequate skin flaps Good skin closure Small to medium sized breasts	As for immediate reconstruction *plus* Well healed scar *plus* No radiotherapy
Myocutaneous flaps	Large skin incision Doubtful skin closure Large breasts	As for immediate reconstruction Can be used if previous radiotherapy

The choice of operation for an individual patient depends on several factors. Immediate breast reconstruction is less time consuming for the patient (though not for the surgeon), but care must be taken that an oncological operation is not jeopardised for a better cosmetic result. Reconstruction can be carried out by immediate placement of a prosthesis (implant), insertion of a tissue expander, or insertion of a flap of skin and muscle (myocutaneous flap) with or without a prosthesis.

Implants and expanders are usually inserted under the chest wall muscles (the pectoralis major and parts of the serratus anterior and rectus abdominis); the expander is inflated over a period of months to stretch the skin and muscle and is eventually replaced with a prosthesis. The two most common myocutaneous flaps used require movement of either the latissimus dorsi muscle with overlying skin or the lower abdominal fat and skin based on the rectus abdominus muscle (transverse rectus abdominus myocutaneous (TRAM) flap). Latissimus flaps usually require a prosthesis to be placed between them and the chest wall to create a breast mound. TRAM flaps—which can be performed as a pedicled flap based on the superior epigastric artery or as a free flap using a microvascular anastomosis—are bulkier and have the great advantage that they do not usually require the insertion of an implant.

All the above reconstructions can give pleasing results in correctly selected patients when performed by experienced surgeons. All forms of breast reconstruction are substantial surgical operations.

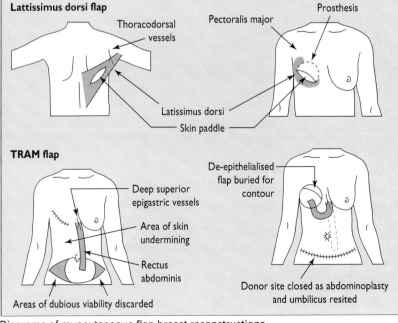

Diagrams of myocutaneous flap breast reconstructions.

Tissue expansion and prostheses

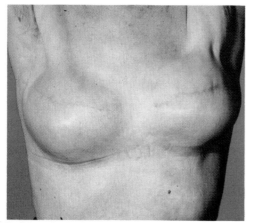

Patient who had immediate placement of bilateral breast prostheses.

The scare about the safety of silicone gel prostheses has put some women off their use. Silicone implants are currently licensed in the United Kingdom and United States for breast reconstructions. Saline prostheses are also available but do not have the same doughy consistency of silicone gel and breast tissue. Prostheses can occasionally provide satisfactory results if inserted immediately at the time of operation or as a delayed procedure in patients with small breasts who have adequate skin flaps. However, prostheses are generally inserted after a period of tissue expansion. Tissue expansion involves placement of a silicone bag connected to a filler port, with saline injected into the filler port at weekly visits. To achieve ptosis of the reconstructed breast, it is necessary to inflate the expander to a greater volume than that of the breast mound to be reconstructed before the expander is replaced with a permanent prosthesis. Tissue expansion is associated with discomfort of the chest wall, and the ribs and chest wall can be substantially depressed immediately under the expander. The development of textured tissue expanders should decrease the prevalence of this discomfort.

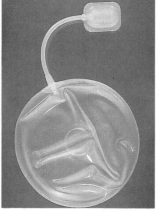

Tissue expander used for breast reconstruction.

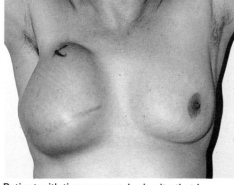

Patient with tissue expander in situ that is overexpanded.

It is difficult to create large breast mounds by tissue expansion. If this technique is to be used in a patient with large breasts the possibility of reducing the contralateral breast should be considered and discussed with the patient. For delayed reconstruction, an expander-prosthesis has recently become available. This contains two cavities, one containing silicone gel and the other which can be inflated with saline. After overinflation the volume of saline is reduced to obtain the desired volume; the filler port is then removed, and the expander-prosthesis is left in situ.

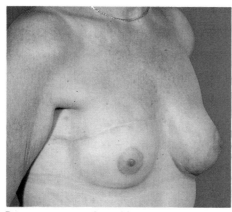

Breast reconstruction with permanent prosthesis after previous tissue expansion. (Nipple complex has also been reconstructed.)

Radiotherapy

Tissue expansion is difficult in patients who have had chest wall radiotherapy and is generally not recommended; radiotherapy causes fibrosis in the chest wall muscles and in the overlying skin, which makes it difficult to obtain satisfactory expansion. In such patients breasts are better reconstructed with a myocutaneous flap. However, patients undergoing tissue expansion or women with a prosthesis in situ can have postoperative chest wall radiotherapy if this is considered appropriate. This should be delivered over a longer period (in a larger number of fractions) than standard schedules to reduce tissue reaction and fibrosis. Chemotherapy can be delivered to patients with prostheses, tissue expanders, or flaps as soon as the wound has healed (areas of skin edge necrosis should preferably have re-epithelialised) and providing there are no signs of underlying infection.

Complications with breast prostheses

Fibrous capsules—The commonest complication after the use of prostheses is the formation and subsequent contraction of fibrous capsules around implants. The use of textured prostheses has reduced the incidence of capsular contraction from over 50% with smooth implants at one year to less than 10%. Capsular contraction results in "hardening" and distortion of the reconstructed breast mound and often causes pain, discomfort, and embarrassment. Possible treatments include closed capsulotomy (forceful manual rupture of the fibrous envelope—the problem is that this can rupture the prosthesis) and capsulectomy or capsulotomy, with change of prosthesis to a textured implant if a smooth implant had been used previously.

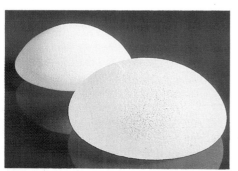

Textured prostheses for breast reconstruction.

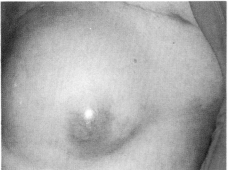

Area of infection over a tissue expander that necessitated removal of the expander.

Saline filled implants are available for breast reconstruction, but early models had a much higher rate of leakage and they produced less satisfactory cosmetic results than silicone filled implants. Prostheses containing non-silicone polymers are now available and are being evaluated.

Infection occurs in about 5% of patients and inevitably results in the prosthesis having to be removed. Most units use prophylactic antibiotics to limit the rate of infection. Low grade infection can occasionally manifest as early capsular contraction or erosion of the prosthesis through the overlying skin.

Implant fatigue and rupture is a major concern among patients as it leads to leakage of silicone gel. About 1% of all implants, in particular earlier varieties with thinner envelopes, are liable to rupture. Ruptured implants seem to cause minimal morbidity. All silicone implants bleed a small amount of silicone gel, but there is no convincing evidence that this is carcinogenic: in a recent Canadian study women who underwent breast augmentation with silicone implants were reported to have a significantly lower rate of subsequent breast cancer than age matched controls. There is also no convincing evidence that the leakage of silicone causes problems in other organs. In particular, women with implants do not seem to have a higher rate of connective tissue disorders (scleroderma, systemic lupus erythematosus, rheumatoid arthritis, etc) than age matched women without implants. Few good studies of this subject have been performed, and research is continuing. The lack of an association between silicone and connective tissue disorders is confirmed by the observation that other patients exposed to silicone (for example, patients with Silastic joints, heart valves containing silicone, or siliconised arteriovenous shunts) do not have an excess of these disorders.

Myocutaneous flap reconstructions

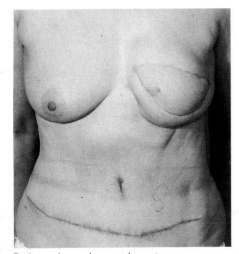

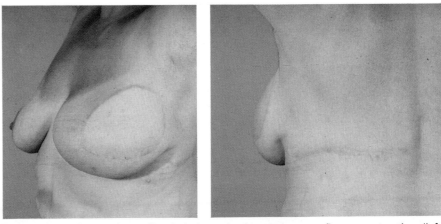

Patient who underwent immediate latissimus dorsi myocutaneous flap reconstruction: (left) side view showing ptosis that can be achieved; (right) scar on back.

Patient who underwent breast reconstruction with TRAM flap; note large abdominal scar.

These have developed over the years from the early "breast sharing" operations to the recent use of free tissue transfer with microvascular anastomoses. In immediate reconstructions with a myocutaneous flap, skin away from the carcinoma can be preserved, which significantly improves the final cosmetic result. Myocutaneous flaps require considerable time and are best performed by two teams of surgeons. Patients for TRAM flaps should be non-smokers and well motivated. Scarring of the donor site and a prolonged recovery period (up to three months after a TRAM flap) must be discussed fully with the patient. With a TRAM flap, the use of lower abdominal skin and fat is often looked on by the patient as a bonus. If it is considered appropriate, radiotherapy can be delivered to the adjacent skin flaps after immediate breast reconstruction with these flaps.

Complications

The greatest problem is flap necrosis. Major necrosis occurs in up to 10% of patients having pedicled TRAM flaps and affects fewer than 5% of patients with free TRAM flaps. It is extremely rare after a latissimus dorsi myocutaneous flap, although minor degrees of necrosis may occur in 5% of patients. Infection can be a problem in latissimus flaps, as an implant is inserted. Removal of the rectus abdominis weakens the abdominal wall, and abdominal hernias occur in about 10% of patients.

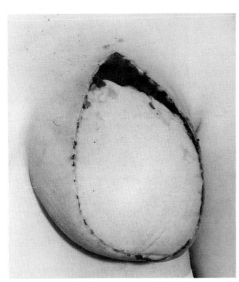

Partial necrosis of upper part of latissimus dorsi myocutaneous flap.

Nipple reconstructions

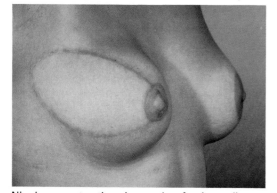

Nipple reconstruction six months after immediate breast reconstruction by latissimus dorsi flap.

In general it is best to wait at least six months after breast reconstruction before reconstructing the nipple complex to allow the breast time to settle. The nipple complex consists of the nipple and the areola, and each is reconstructed by different methods.

The areola

Dark skin for the new areola can be obtained from the upper inner thigh, or in some situations part of the contralateral areola can be used. In experienced hands tattooing can recreate the areola, but the colour intensity of the tattooed areola fades with time so the procedure may have to be repeated.

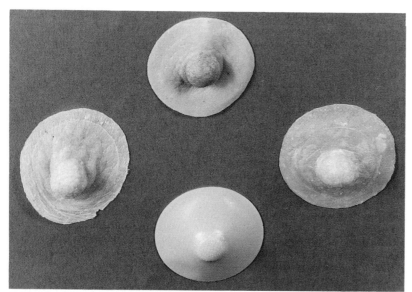

Customised prosthetic nipple (top) and commercially available ones.

The nipple

Several techniques have been devised to make use of local tissue to produce nipple prominence. When the contralateral nipple is particularly prominent, "nipple sharing" is a possibility.

Use of prosthetic nipples—A false nipple can give a satisfactory shape and colour. An impression is made of the remaining nipple, and a colour matched silicone nipple is prepared by the lost wax technique. This can be prepared in a dental laboratory in two or three days. Patients apply the nipples with medical adhesive and wear them for a month at a time, thereafter peeling them off to wash the skin underneath.

Reduction mammoplasty and mastopexy

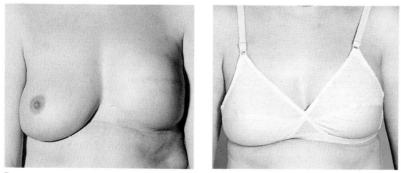

Breast reconstruction with tissue expansion and prosthesis: lack of ptosis in reconstructed breast (left), which is hidden when a bra is worn (right).

It is not always possible to reconstruct a breast mound that matches the natural breast. Both size and shape can pose problems. Major problems with breast reconstructions are that they sit high and proud and often display little in the way of ptosis. If a good match of breast volume has been achieved this lack of ptosis can be hidden by a good bra, thus achieving symmetry when the patient is fully clothed. Some women are happy with this, while others wish to have the contralateral breast lifted surgically by mastopexy.

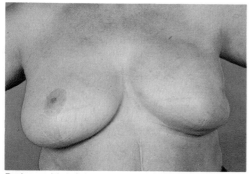

Patient with left breast reconstruction by tissue expansion and prosthesis; she subsequently had right breast reduced to achieve symmetry.

When there is a substantial difference in size, symmetry (even when clothed) can only be achieved by reduction of the natural breast. Some women who have chosen to wear an external prosthesis after a mastectomy and who have no interest in breast reconstruction may seek reduction of their remaining breast to allow them to wear a smaller and lighter prosthesis.

Complications

These operations can produce considerable permanent scarring, which can be of a variable quality. Delayed skin healing, skin and nipple necrosis, change in or loss of nipple sensation, and an inability to breast feed are specific problems related to reduction mammoplasty and mastopexy.

Other operations

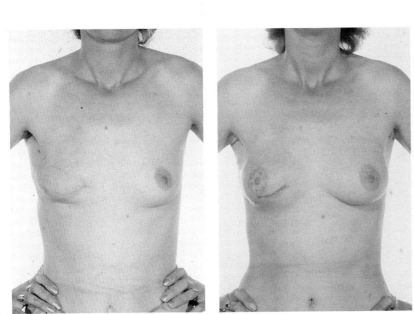

Patient who had right breast reconstruction by latissimus dorsi flap with small implant underneath (left). Subsequently, both reconstructed and normal breast were enlarged at patient's request and a nipple reconstruction was performed to achieve better cosmetic result (right).

Augmentation mammoplasty after contralateral breast reconstruction

Occasionally, in women with small breasts the reconstructed side may be larger than their natural breast. This can be corrected by augmenting the unoperated side with a prosthesis filled with silicone gel or saline. Some women take the opportunity of breast reconstruction to achieve larger breasts.

Reconstruction after wide local excision

There have been attempts to improve the cosmetic outcome after wide local excision by means of prostheses or myocutaneous flaps. Such techniques are necessary only when extensive excisions have been performed. Few published results are available to determine whether these techniques do produce satisfactory cosmetic results.

Breast cancer after cosmetic breast augmentation

Patients who develop breast cancer after breast augmentation can be treated either by breast conserving treatment (wide local excision and breast radiotherapy) if their lesion is appropriate for this approach or by mastectomy. Radiotherapy given to an augmented breast should be delivered over a longer period to reduce tissue reaction and fibrosis around the prosthesis, optimising the final cosmetic result. For women who require a mastectomy, symmetry can be achieved by immediate breast reconstruction.

INDEX

Index

Index

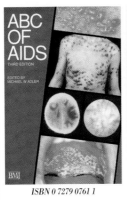
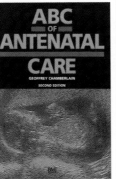
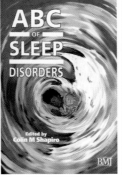
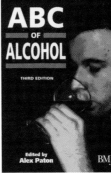
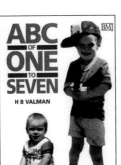
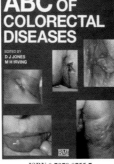
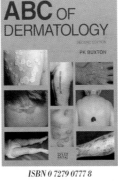
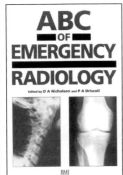
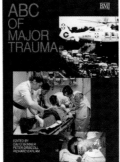
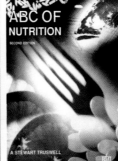
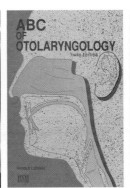
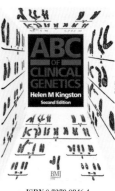
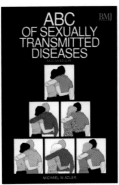
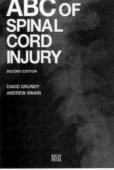
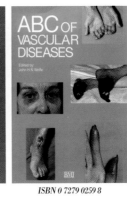
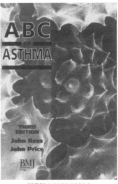
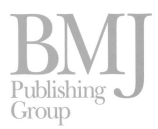